NURSES' GUIDE TO CARDIA

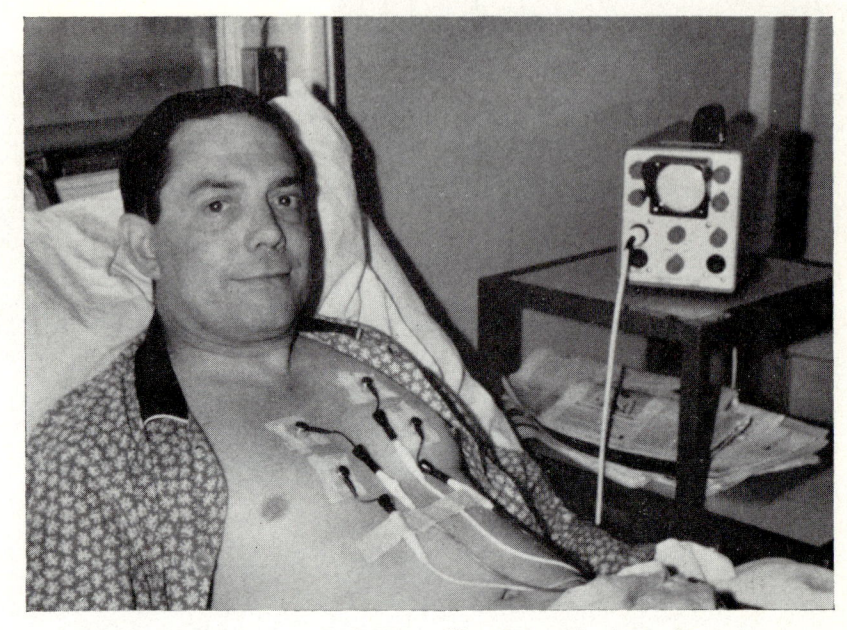

Patient connected to an ECG oscilloscope with chest electrodes.

NURSES' GUIDE TO
Cardiac monitoring

P. J. B. Hubner, M.B., M.R.C.P.
Cardiology Registrar, Royal Postgraduate Medical School,
Hammersmith Hospital, London

WITH A FOREWORD BY

Professor **J. P. Shillingford**, M.D., F.R.C.P.
Professor of Angiocardiology, Honorary Consultant
Physician to Hammersmith Hospital, and Director of
the M.R.C. Cardiovascular Research Unit

BAILLIÈRE TINDALL · LONDON

First published 1971
Reprinted 1972

Copyright © 1971

Baillière, Tindall & Cassell Ltd
7 & 8 Henrietta Street, London W.C.2

ISBN 0 7020 0378 6

Published in the United States of America
by the Williams & Wilkins Company, Baltimore

Made and printed in Great Britain by Headley Brothers Ltd
109 Kingsway London WC2 and Ashford Kent

Foreword

THE last decade has seen a remarkable advance in the treatment of patients following myocardial infarction. The introduction of external cardiac massage, respiratory support, the direct current defibrillator, and pacing of the heart have all contributed to this advance. At the same time there has been considerable development in the introduction of new and powerful anti-arrhythmic remedies. The introduction of the concept of intensive coronary care, where the patient is kept under constant observation with the facilities for the treatment of arrhythmias or other complications as they occur, has reduced the mortality of patients entering hospital from over 30 per cent to approximately 15 to 20 per cent.

These developments have meant, however, that it is now necessary to train a new generation of nurses and physicians in the rapid interpretation of the electrocardiographic records together with constant observation of the patient and knowledge of the complications following myocardial infarction as they occur. This small paperback produced by Dr Hubner, who has had considerable experience working in the pioneer intensive care unit in a teaching hospital, and also in peripheral hospitals, will come as a welcome aid to nurses and housemen alike responsible for the care of patients in coronary care units, and will serve as a stepping stone for those who may be interested to read further into this important subject.

There is no doubt that over the next few years many further advances will be made in the management of patients seriously ill following myocardial infarction, and for this reason it is desirable that a handbook of this type should be kept small and in a form that can easily be modified in further editions.

February 1971   PROFESSOR J. P. SHILLINGFORD

Preface

This book has been derived from the lectures on cardiac monitoring given to the nurses of the coronary care and surgical intensive care units at the Royal Postgraduate Medical School, Hammersmith Hospital. The purpose of cardiac monitoring and origin of the normal electrocardiogram (ECG) trace are explained. The application of electrodes to the patient and the basic features and controls of monitors are described, together with the methods for observing a monitor screen to detect whether the ECG trace is normal or is showing an arrhythmia. The majority of the common arrhythmias are listed and their significances given; also included is a section on the monitor traces of satisfactory and disturbed cardiac pacing.

Several of the more sophisticated aspects of monitors and arrhythmias have been omitted. Although simple and sometimes less precise terms are used, care has been taken to avoid inaccuracies. The emphasis throughout is on what the nurse observes on the monitor screen. For this reason the method of recording a standard ECG on an ECG machine, and the interpretation of wave forms in the diagnosis of cardiac conditions such as myocardial infarction and pulmonary embolism, have been excluded. It is not considered the nurse's duty to diagnose these conditions, but rather to recognize arrhythmias which may result from them.

Besides the ECG, cardiac patients may have other parameters monitored, such as central venous pressure. Following cardiac surgery, patients may require artificial respiration with a ventilator. These topics and the nurse's duty in general, for patients receiving intensive care, are not discussed because they are adequately covered in existing textbooks.

Stress has been laid on the fact that the patient must always come first and that monitor observation is always subsidiary to the care and observation of the patient. However, as the ECG is becoming more and more frequently monitored, nurses do need to know how the equipment is used and what the ECG trace on the monitor screen is showing.

It is with great pleasure that I acknowledge the assistance given to me in the preparation of this book by the many nurses that I have taught. I am very grateful to Professor J. P. Shillingford for kindly writing the Foreword. I also wish to thank Dr M. J. Goldberg and Mr P. A. Burgess for their advice and encouragement, Miss J. Powell for the preparation of the diagrams, and Cambridge Scientific Instruments Ltd and Cardiac Recorders Ltd for technical illustrations.

P.J.B.H.

*This small book is dedicated to
my wife, my parents, N.D.L. and M.J.G.*

Contents

FOREWORD		v
PREFACE		vii
CHAPTER 1	The monitors	1
CHAPTER 2	Electrodes	7
CHAPTER 3	The normal ECG trace	11
CHAPTER 4	The arrhythmias. I. Sinus brachycardia, sinus tachycardia and extrasystoles	19
CHAPTER 5	The arrhythmias. II. Atrial and ventricular tachycardia, atrial flutter and atrial fibrillation	29
CHAPTER 6	The arrhythmias. III. Heart block	35
CHAPTER 7	Cardiac arrest	43
CHAPTER 8	Cardiac pacing	45
CHAPTER 9	General notes and hints on monitor observation	55
INDEX		63

CHAPTER 1

The monitors

Cardiac monitoring with electrocardiograph (ECG) oscilloscopes is often used routinely in the management of patients after a myocardial infarction, after cardiac surgery, and following resuscitation from cardiac arrest. The reason for monitoring is to detect and then treat *disturbances of rhythm of the heart beat*. These disturbances (termed 'arrhythmias') may impair the heart's pumping action and may herald or cause cessation of the heart beat, i.e. a cardiac arrest. Patients with pacemakers (machines used to speed up certain types of slow heart rate) are frequently monitored to determine whether pacing is satisfactory.

Nurses are more and more frequently caring for patients connected to monitors. They must, therefore, know how to attach electrodes and operate the monitors. They should be able to appreciate the normal and recognize the abnormal traces displayed on the screen of a monitor. With this knowledge nurses need not feel anxious in the presence of monitors. More important, however, they will be able to detect arrhythmias and thus actively help in the management of the patient.

The normal nurse–patient relationship need not be disturbed just because the patient is connected to a piece of electronic apparatus from which the nurse makes observations, as well as from the patient himself. The care and observation of the patient must always take preference over that of the monitor. This principle, however, is no excuse for the total neglect of monitor observation.

Nurses should take the time to inform the patient and the relatives that though the heart is being monitored, this does not necessarily mean that the patient is critically ill. It should be explained that the patient is having the benefit of the most up-to-date medical care to speed the recovery. In this way, anxiety of patients and their relatives will be reduced or avoided altogether.

Aim of Cardiac Monitoring

The chief purpose of monitoring is to *confirm that the heart rhythm is normal* or to *detect that the heart rhythm is abnormal*, i.e. an arrhythmia is present.

Indications for Cardiac Monitoring with ECG Oscilloscopes

1. After acute myocardial infarction
2. During and after surgery especially cardiac
3. After cardiac arrest
4. During cardiac catheterization

} to detect disturbances of the heart beat (arrhythmias).

5. Patients with arrhythmias—to assess progress during treatment.
6. Patients with pacemakers—to determine whether pacing is satisfactory.

Components for Cardiac Monitoring

There are two components for cardiac monitoring: the *cardiac monitor* on which the ECG trace is displayed, and the *electrodes* which make

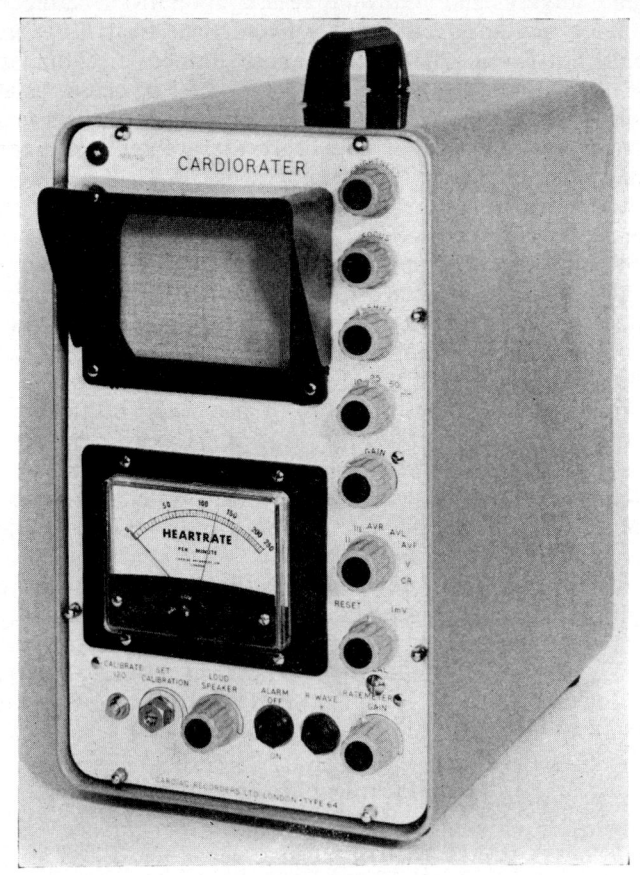

FIG. 1. Cardiac monitor (Cardiac Recorders Ltd).

THE MONITORS 3

contact with the patient allowing electricity flowing from the patient with each heart beat to pass along to the monitor.
Monitors (synonyms: cardiac monitors, ECG oscilloscopes, 'scopes).

These pieces of equipment are like small television sets on which the heart beat trace (electrocardiogram, ECG) is displayed (Figs 1 and 2).

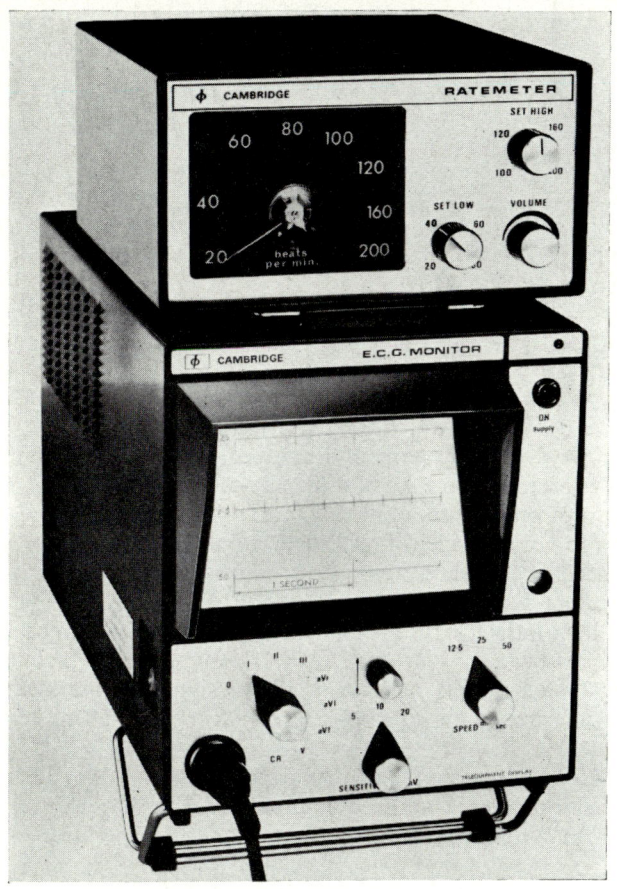

FIG. 2. Cardiac monitor (Cambridge Scientific Instruments Ltd).

There are a wide variety of monitors of varying complexity. Most monitors (Fig. 3) have in common:
1. *Mains cable:* has a plug which is inserted into the mains socket to supply electricity to operate the monitor.

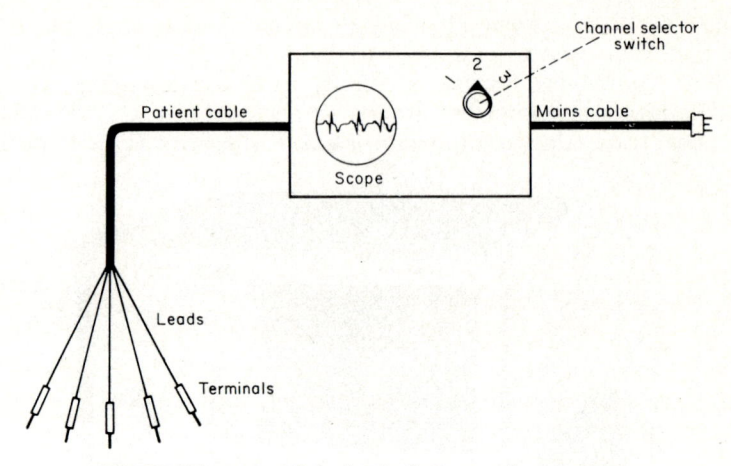

Fig. 3. Diagram of the basic features of a monitor.

2. *Patient cable:* divides into three to five often coloured wires (called *leads*) with terminals which connect to the electrodes on the patient.
3. *Scope or screen:* on which the ECG trace is displayed.
4. *Selector switch:* allows one of a number of channels to be used so that the one selected offers the best display of the ECG trace.

Other features on monitors may include:
(a) Knobs to control size (often called 'gain'), brightness, focus, position and speed of the trace.
(b) Ratemeter: displaying the heart rate.
(c) Heart beat indicator: a sound ('bleep') or a flashing light occurs with each heart beat.
(d) Alarm system: emits audible or visual signals if the heart rate falls below or exceeds an adjustable preset level, e.g. 50 to 110 beats per min.
(e) Record system: a short strip of paper on which the ECG is written starts automatically at fixed intervals (e.g. every 30 min), or when the alarm system operates, or when a button is pressed.

Practical Points about Monitors

The monitor should not be camouflaged behind flowers, get-well cards, etc., in the hope that everyone will forget about it! Preferably have the monitor on its own separate table or trolley. If it is placed on top of the patient's locker, have nothing else on top with it.

Controls: The only way to become accustomed to the monitors used in

THE MONITORS 5

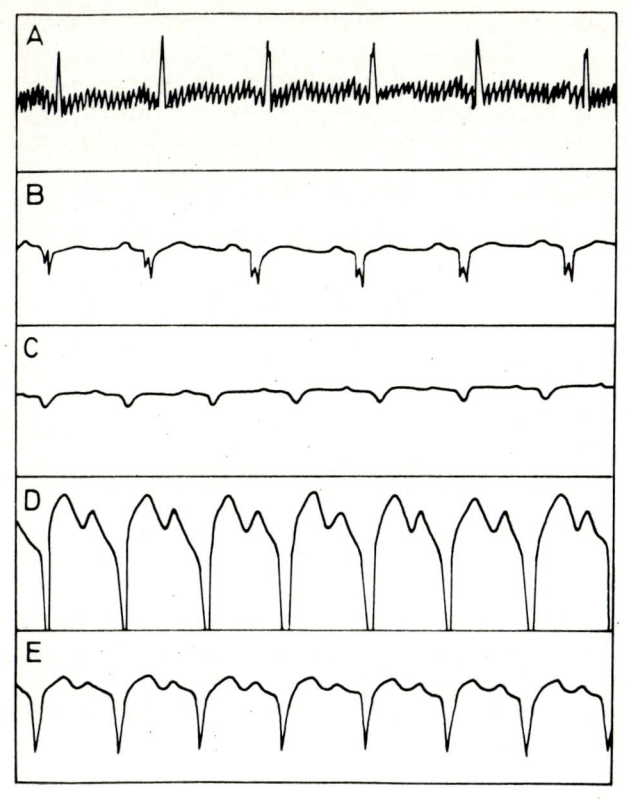

ECG 1. (A) 'fuzzy' (interference) trace, corrected to (B) by selecting a different monitor channel. (C), (D) and (E) are the same trace with complexes too small (C), too large (D), and of the correct size (E).

the ward is to ask the house-doctor, sister or staff-nurse to demonstrate the various controls. Subsequently, alter the knobs one at a time yourself to see and learn the action of each.

Brightness: Always use the minimum brightness necessary to see the trace. If the trace is surrounded by a ring as it travels across the screen, it is too bright. At night as the ward is dark, less brightness is required. Attention to these points will help to prolong the working life of the monitor. On altering brightness refocusing may be necessary.

Channel: Select the channel (Fig. 4, ECG 1A–E): (a) which shows the trace as a thin line as opposed to a thick fuzzy one which will obscure the smaller waves (ECG 1A and 20B); and (b) which shows the waves of the trace clearly, i.e. waves which are not too small. It may be necessary to increase the size of the waves by adjusting the appropriate knob (which is sometimes called 'gain'). Usually it does not matter what shape or direction (upright or inverted) the waves have, as long as they are clearly identifiable.

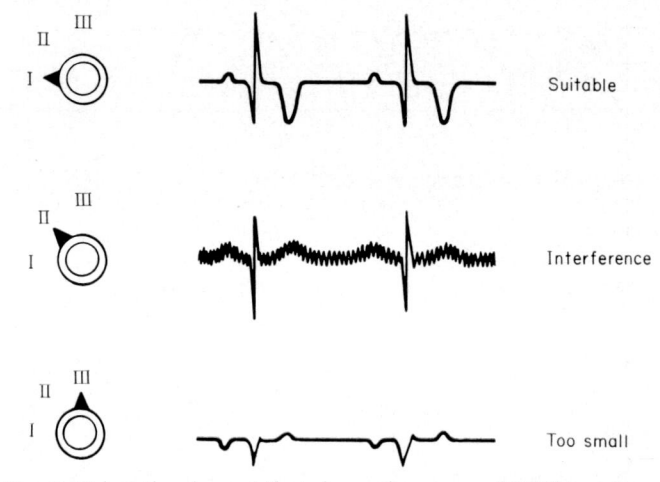

FIG. 4. Select the channel that shows the waves of ECG trace most clearly.

CHAPTER 2

Electrodes

Electrodes allow contact between the skin and the leads of the patient cable which passes to the monitor. Electricity flowing from the patient with each heart beat is thus able to travel to the monitor and be displayed on the monitor screen as the ECG trace.

Electrodes are metal plates which may be placed on either the limbs or on the chest.

LIMB ELECTRODES

Limb electrodes (Fig. 5) are flat metal plates, which have on their top side a socket into which the lead terminal of the patient cable is secured, usually by a screw. The electrode is strapped to the patient by a band of rubber passing round the limb. One electrode is placed on each limb, usually above the wrist or ankle, though any position on the limb can be used. On the legs the electrode must be placed on the outer (lateral) side,

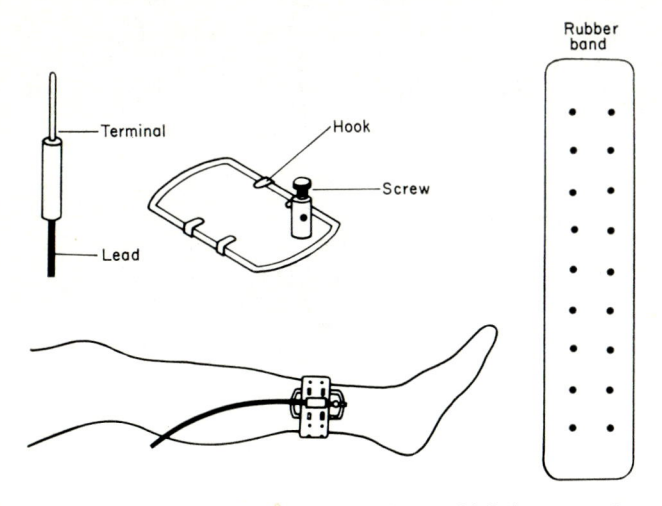

FIG. 5. Limb electrodes—flat metal plates which have on the top side a socket into which the lead terminal of the patient cable is secured.

so that with the screw facing outwards, scratching of the opposite leg on the screw is avoided. Before using a limb electrode ensure its surface is clean and not covered with green crusts, as these will produce a poor trace and may cause skin reactions. After their use wipe the surfaces clean with a paper tissue or piece of gauze. Dirty electrodes covered with crusts can be cleaned with methylated spirits or ether; sometimes rubbing the surface with fine sandpaper may be required.

CHEST ELECTRODES

As these electrodes are placed on the chest, movements of the limbs are not restricted and produce less interference to the ECG trace on the screen. The standard limb electrodes may be strapped to the chest, but preferably special chest electrodes are used. Each consists of a small metal disc or piece of metal gauze with an arrangement to secure it to the chest. Two examples of chest electrodes, and the method of attachment of the lead to the electrode are shown in Fig. 6.

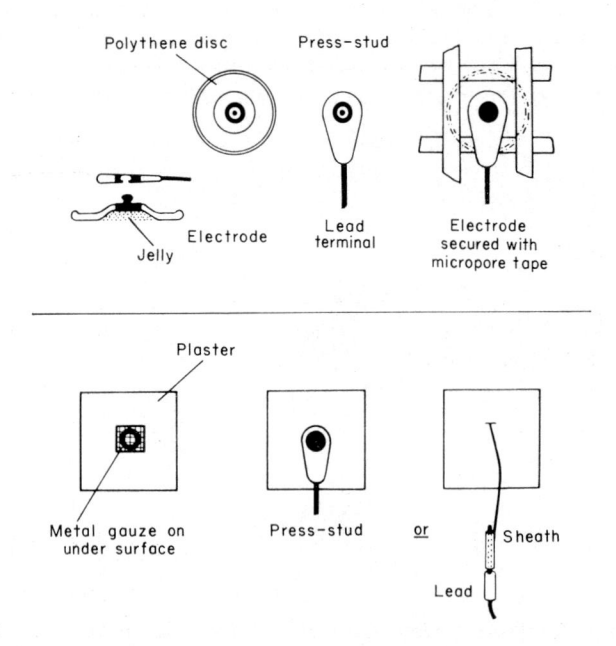

FIG. 6. Two types of chest electrode and their method of lead attachment to the electrode.

ELECTRODES

Position of Chest Electrodes

The exact position of chest electrodes is unimportant. Surgical wounds will preclude certain sites. They may be positioned down the sternum, or along the side of it, below the nipple area, or under the clavicles (Fig. 7). In women with pendulous breasts, electrodes may be placed on or above, but not under the breasts because at this last site skin excoriation may

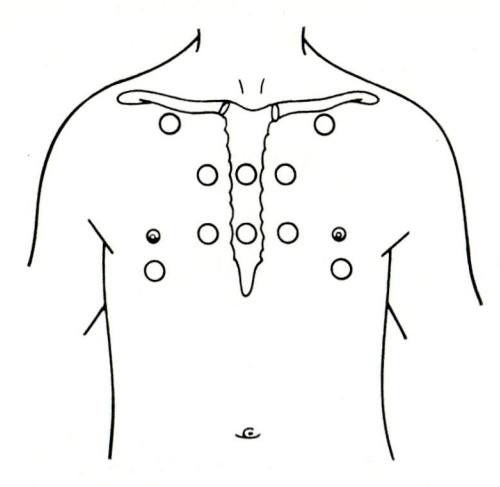

FIG. 7. Chest electrode sites: along either side of the sternum; down the sternum; under the nipples; under the clavicles.

occur. Three or four electrodes are usually employed. Sometimes electrodes may have to be moved around to obtain a satisfactory trace, i.e. a thin one (free of 'fuzzy' interference, ECG 1A, p. 5), showing waves of an adequate size.

APPLICATION OF ELECTRODES (LIMB OR CHEST) TO SKIN

1. Shave hair from proposed sites (not necessary for limb electrodes).
2. Clean skin *carefully and thoroughly* at electrode sites to remove grease. Grease from the natural skin oils increases the resistance to flow of electricity from the patient to the electrode, or in other words, it produces a poor electrical contact. With chest electrodes skin cleaning is a particularly important step as the size of the metal contact is much smaller than with the limb electrodes (see Figs 5 and 6). Using a piece of gauze or a tissue paper soaked with ether (or ether–meths, alcohol or

acetone), rub the skin five to ten times till mild redness (erythema) of the skin appears. Allow skin to dry.

3. *Apply a non-irritant jelly to the electrode.* K-Y jelly (Johnson & Johnson) is suitable and usually readily available. There are other preparations, some especially designed for monitoring, e.g. Cambridge monitoring electrode jelly, coming in *blue* tubes. Cambridge electrode jelly, coming in *yellow* tubes and commonly used for standard ECGs, must not be used as its high salt content produces skin reactions on long term monitoring. With chest electrodes, do not smother the electrode with jelly, otherwise some of it will spill over on to the plaster or adhesive and impair the attachment of the electrode to the skin.

4. Apply the electrodes to limb or chest.

5. Connect terminals of the leads from patient cable to the electrodes. In general, it is not important that any particular lead of the patient cable is connected to any particular electrode.

6. Secure the leads of the monitor cable. To avoid any strain on the leads being transmitted to chest electrodes, the leads should be secured to the skin of the lower chest or upper abdomen with Micropore tape (3M Company) or with plaster.

'Fuzzy Trace'—Interference Pattern

A satisfactory trace is a thin one travelling across the monitor screen at the same level. The fuzzy interference trace (Fig. 4, ECGs 1A and 20B) obscures the P and T waves. The most frequent reason for obtaining this type of trace on applying the electrodes is inadequate skin cleaning. In particular, it is important that ether or one of the other fat solvents mentioned above, should be used to remove skin grease. If this trace is obtained after applying the electrodes, before taking them all off and starting again, it is worth while carrying out the steps suggested on p. 56, as there may be a simpler and quicker remedy.

Replacement of Electrodes

Electrodes may be removed routinely after a given period of 1 to 7 days. In general, the longer an electrode is on at one site the greater the chance of a skin reaction.

Electrodes should be changed and repositioned if: (a) the electrode is obviously loose and about to become displaced; (b) there is irritation of the skin at the electrode site; and (c) the trace is no longer satisfactory, i.e. obscured by 'fuzzy' interference, other methods to improve the trace having failed (see p. 56). Attention to the electrodes should be a daily nursing duty comparable to that of the care of pressure areas.

CHAPTER 3

The normal ECG trace

Anatomy and Physiology

To understand the trace displayed on the scope it is necessary to: (a) appreciate the basic anatomy of the heart and circulation; and (b) to know the origin and pathway of the impulse stimulating the heart to contract.

Blood returning along the veins from the tissues of the body, passes via the superior and inferior vena cavae to enter the right atrium (Fig. 8).

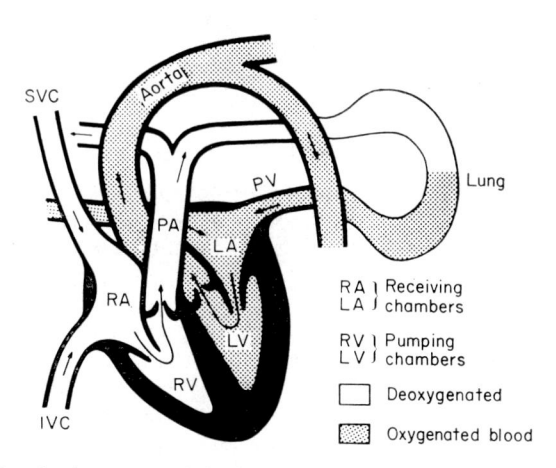

FIG. 8. Anatomy of the heart and course of the blood.

It next crosses the tricuspid valve in to the right ventricle, from where it is pumped out across the pulmonary valve to the pulmonary artery and thence to the lungs. In the lungs the blood is oxygenated and carbon dioxide is given off. Blood returns from the lungs via the pulmonary veins to reach the left atrium. It then crosses the mitral valve to the left ventricle, from where it is pumped across the aortic valve to the aorta, and along the arteries to arrive at the tissues of the body. For a more detailed description of the heart and circulation standard textbooks should be consulted.

It is a characteristic of heart muscle to contract rhythmically, even if the heart is completely removed from the body. Normally however, heart muscle contracts and the heart 'beats' in response to a stimulus, which arises as an impulse from the *sino-atrial (SA) node* (Fig. 9). This is a small C-shaped structure about 2·5 cm (1 in.) long in the wall of the right

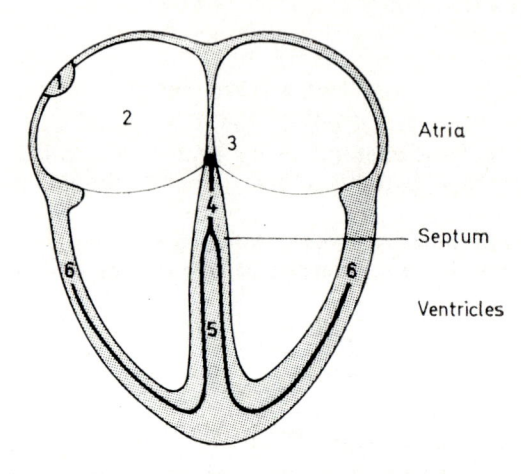

FIG. 9. Origin and conduction of impulse stimulating contraction of heart muscle. 1, SA node; 2, spread of impulse through atria; 3, AV node; 4, Bundle of His; 5, left and right branches of Bundle of His; 6, ventricle muscle.

atrium near the entrance of the superior vena cava. Impulses arise spontaneously from the SA node at the rate of approximately 70 per min, that is the normal resting pulse rate. The rate may be reduced by parasympathetic stimulation (via the vagus nerve), or increased by sympathetic stimulation (by sympathetic nerves or by adrenaline circulating in the blood stream).

From the SA node the impulse spreads through the atria, like ripples spread from a pebble dropped into water, stimulating atrial contraction. The impulse next reaches the *atrio-ventricular (AV) node*, which is situated near the tricuspid valve. There is a short hold-up or delay to conduction of the impulse whilst it crosses the AV node. The impulse next passes down the *Bundle of His* which divides after a short length into left and right branches. The impulse arriving at the end of the ramifications of the bundle branches, activates the ventricular muscle which then contracts. The Bundle of His and its branches are composed of special muscle fibres (called Purkinje fibres) which allow rapid conduction of the impulse.

THE NORMAL ECG TRACE

The course of events may be summarized (Fig. 9):
1. Impulse originates from SA node.
2. Impulse spreads across atria causing their contraction.
3. Impulse arrives at AV node.
4. Impulse passes down the Bundle of His.
5. Impulse passes along the Bundle branches.
6. Impulse arrives at the ventricular muscles which then contract.

Now follows a period of heart rest after which an impulse again arises at the SA node and follows the same pathway from the atria to the ventricles.

The normal rhythm of the heart, with initial impulse arising from the SA node, is referred to as *sinus rhythm*. The SA node which produces the impulses, is known as the *pacemaker* of the heart.

The Normal ECG trace

The normal ECG trace is displayed in Fig. 10.

P wave: represents electrical activity associated with an impulse arising from the SA node producing atrial contraction.

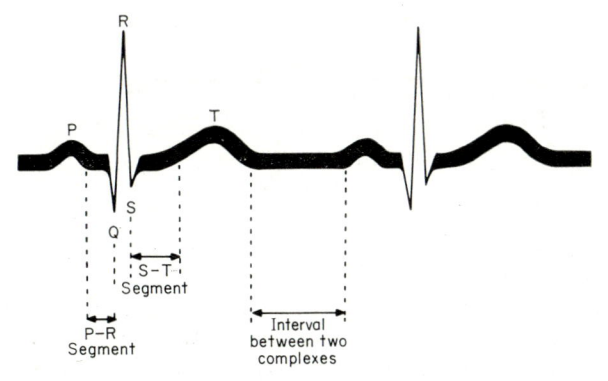

FIG. 10. Normal ECG trace. P wave + QRS complex + T wave = one complex. QRS complex + T wave = one QRS–T complex.

P–R Segment: from the end of the P wave to the start of the QRS complex. It represents conduction of the impulse across AV node, and down the bundle of His and its branches to the ventricular muscle.

QRS complex: represents electrical activity associated with ventricular contraction.

T wave: represents the electrical activity associated with the onset of ventricular relaxation.

After the T wave, there follows the period of heart rest and the trace shows a straight line till the cycle is repeated with the next P wave. Usually no wave is seen on the ECG trace representing atrial relaxation, as its timing coincides with ventricular contraction, so that it is obscured by the QRS complex.

The S–T segment: is from the end of the QRS complex to the beginning of the T wave.

The P wave plus the QRS complex and T wave are collectively known as *one complex*.

The QRS complex (ventricular contraction) is always followed by a T wave (ventricular relaxation). The QRS complex and T wave should, therefore, be thought of as one unit, which may be referred to as the '*QRS–T complex*'.

Sometimes a small extra wave may clearly be seen at the end of the T wave; it is called a '*U wave*' (Fig. 11, ECG 21C). Its origin is uncertain. Its importance lies in not confusing it with an extra (and abnormal) P wave.

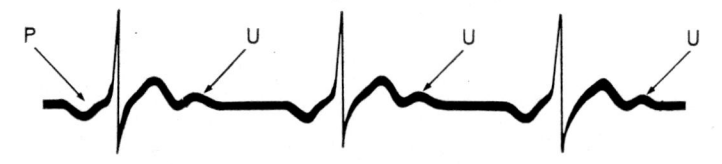

FIG. 11. The U wave.

The shape, size and direction (upright or inverted) of a P wave or QRS–T complex are collectively known as the *configuration* of the wave or complex. Provided that the configuration is constant, the configuration particularly the direction, is not important with monitoring. Though both heart diseases and arrhythmias influence whether the P and T waves and QRS complexes are upright or inverted, their direction is also dependent upon the siting of the electrodes and the channel selected for monitoring.

The P–R segment is from the end of the P wave to the beginning of the QRS–T complex. This term must not be mistaken for the *P–R interval* which rather confusingly is defined as the distance from the *beginning* of the P wave to the beginning of the QRS–T complex.

The Three Rules for Monitor Observation

Monitor observation is not difficult if one knows how and what to look for.

THE NORMAL ECG TRACE   15

1. Observe the Monitor Frequently

The exact frequency of monitor observation depends on the reason for monitoring and whether any arrhythmia is displayed. Within reason, the more frequently the monitor is observed the better; however never neglect the observation of the patient which *must* always take preference over monitor observation. Whenever practical do not walk past a monitor without stopping to observe the trace.

2. Observe the Monitor Sufficiently

Don't just glance at one or two complexes. Observe all the complexes as the trace travels across the monitor screen on six successive occasions; for very large monitor screens (23 cm [9 in.] diameter and larger) this figure may be reduced to three.

3. Observe the Monitor Carefully

Observe the trace carefully for four features.

(a) P wave	Present or absent.
(b) QRS–T complex	Ensure each is preceded by a P wave. Attempt to assess whether the length of the P–R segment is normal or prolonged. Constant or varying shape to QRS–T complexes.
(c) Heart rate	Fast, slow or normal. Regular or irregular.
(d) Extras	Any extra P waves or QRS–T complexes.

The exact configuration of the P wave and QRS–T complex is not important unless it is varying. It is the rhythm, not shape, that is all important with ECG monitoring. The number and width of the complexes as the trace travels across the screen depends on the heart rate and the speed of the trace. With 7·5 to 10 cm (3 to 4 in.) diameter screens adjust the speed so that with sinus rhythm at a normal heart rate (70 to 100/min) between four to six complexes will appear as the ECG trace travels across the screen.

With monitor observation the P–R segment should be considered to 'belong' to the QRS–T complex. Whenever looking at a QRS–T complex, determine whether a P wave precedes it and whether the P–R segment is normal or prolonged. This assessment of the P–R segment length

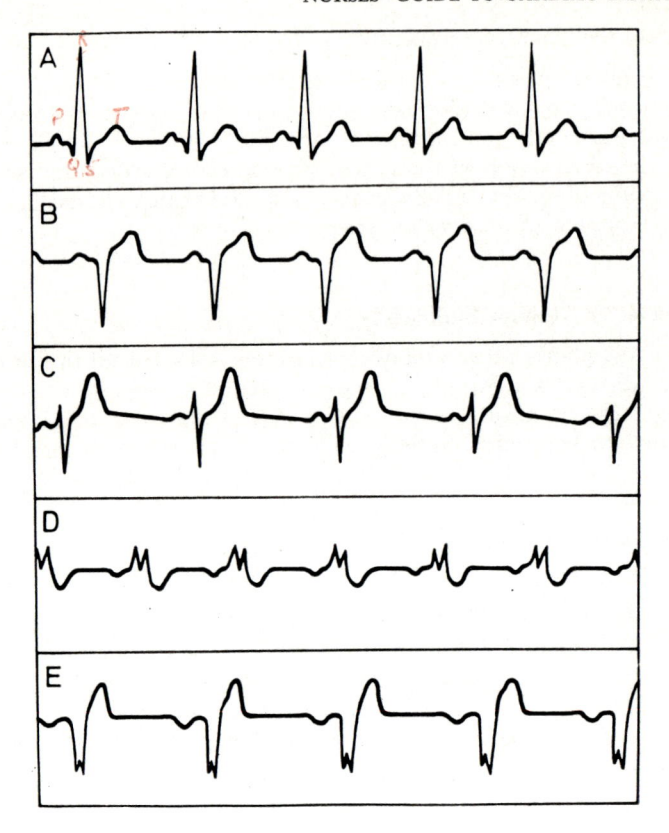

ECG 2. (A)–(E) are examples of normal traces, i.e. sinus rhythm at a normal rate.

though difficult at first, should be attempted and will become easier with experience.

By assessing the distance (gap) between spikes of successive QRS–T complexes, with practice it is possible to detect whether the heart rate is fast, slow, or about normal, and whether it is regular or irregular. If the distance is large or small the rate is slow or fast respectively; if the distance is constant or varying, the rate is regular or irregular respectively. One's opinion may be confirmed by feeling the pulse.

ECG 2A–E are examples of normal traces, i.e. ECG traces showing sinus rhythm at a normal heart rate. The wide variety in configuration of the P waves and QRS–T complexes of traces which do not show an arrhythmia may be seen. On each set of ECGs 3–16 and 20–22, the top panel is devoted to an example of a trace showing sinus rhythm at a normal heart rate.

CHAPTER 4

The arrhythmias

I. Sinus brachycardia, sinus tachycardia and extrasystoles

The main purpose of cardiac monitoring is to detect rhythm disturbances of the heart (arrhythmias) and assess their treatment. There are a very large number of arrhythmias, some more important than others. Some are difficult to assess from the monitor and require a formal ECG to be taken.

The arrhythmias which will be discussed are: (a) those more easily recognized on the monitor screen, and/or (b) those of practical importance.

The importance of arrhythmia will in part be dependent upon the underlying heart condition, i.e. the reason for monitoring. Classification of arrhythmias by their importance will, therefore, not be made. Nor will a classification be attempted by the supposed underlying mechanism or site at fault, as these are complicated, not fully understood, and not particularly helpful in the recognition of arrhythmias from the scope.

SINUS BRADYCARDIA AND SINUS TACHYCARDIA

These are, respectively, slow and fast regular heart rates, (brady — slow, tachy — fast). They are normal inasmuch as the stimulating impulse arises from the SA node. The heart rate is 60 or less, and 110 or more per min in sinus bradycardia and sinus tachycardia, respectively.

On the Monitor (ECG 3B–E)

	Sinus bradycardia	*Sinus tachycardia*
P wave	Present.	Present.
QRS–T complex	Each preceded by a P wave.	Each preceded by a P wave.
	P–R segment normal.	P–R segment normal.
	QRS–T shape constant.	QRS–T shape constant.
Heart rate	*Slow*, regular.	*Fast*, regular.
Extras	None.	None.

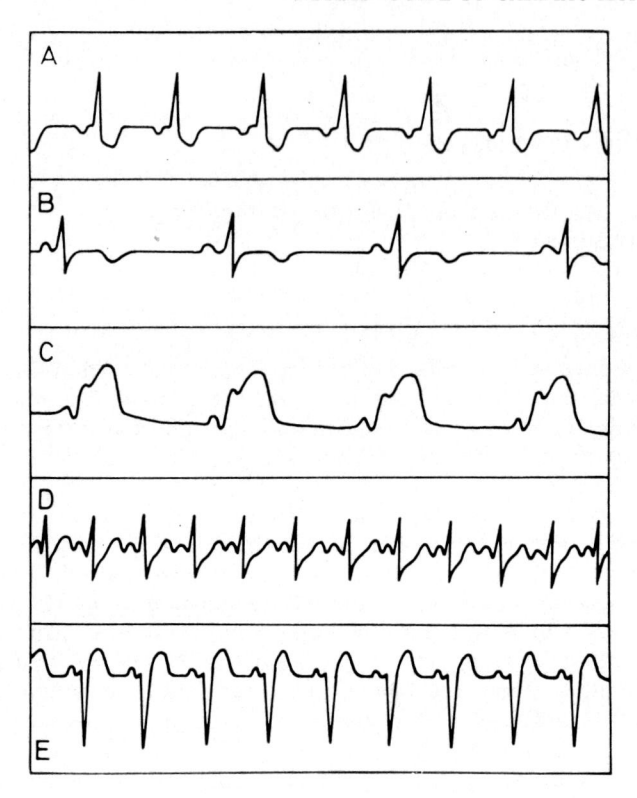

ECG 3. (A) sinus rhythm at normal heart rate; (B) and (C) sinus bradycardia; (D) and (E) sinus tachycardia.

Significance of Sinus Bradycardia and Sinus Tachycardia

Sinus bradycardia is not usually serious; in fact, it is the slow heart rate possessed by very fit athletes! It may occur after acute myocardial infarction, particularly after the administration of morphine or pethidine for analgesia. In this situation sinus bradycardia may lead to a fall of blood pressure, and more rarely even to loss of consciousness. If hypotension occurs, the foot of the bed should be raised and atropine may be given, usually intravenously. Atropine increases the heart rate by blocking the slowing action of the vagus nerve in the discharge of impulses from the SA node. The slow heart rate of a fainting episode (vasovagal attack) is sinus bradycardia.

Sinus tachycardia is the fast heart rate occurring on exercise, with anxiety, with fever, during severe haemorrhage, and in thyrotoxicosis. It is a feature of acute heart failure, particularly after myocardial infarction. It is the fast heart rate (120 to 160 per min) possessed by normal neonates. Sinus tachycardia is not in itself important, because its heart rate is not very fast (100 to 140 per min), and also because it is not a disturbed cardiac rhythm, but often merely a compensatory reaction to an event (e.g. a haemorrhage) which has occurred outside the heart. Hence no treatment is required for sinus tachycardia itself, but correction of an underlying cause may be necessary.

EXTRASYSTOLE OR ECTOPIC BEAT

An extrasystole is also known as an ectopic beat ('ectopic'), a premature ventricular contraction (PVC) or a premature ventricular beat (PVB). An extrasystole is one of the most important rhythm disturbances to detect by monitor observation.

An extrasystole is an *extra*, usually earlier, ventricular contraction, whose stimulating impulse has not arisen from the SA node, but from an abnormal or ectopic site. (An ectopic pregnancy is one outside the womb.) The synonyms for extrasystoles will help in remembering these features:

1. extra   extrasystole
2. earlier ventricular contraction   premature ventricular contraction
3. whose stimulating impulse arises
   from an abnormal (ectopic) site   ectopic beat

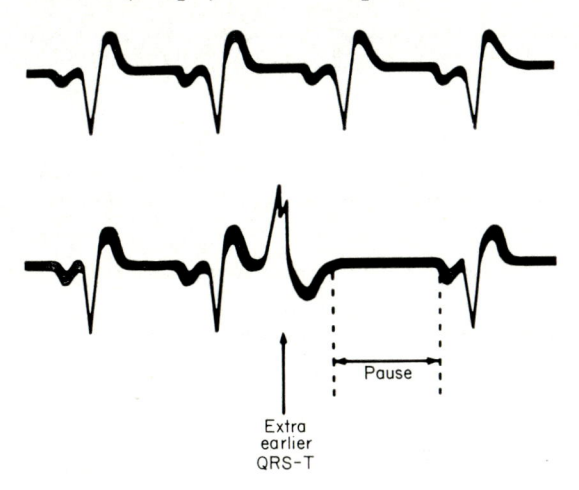

FIG. 12. ECG showing extrasystole which is seen as an earlier QRS–T complex.

On the Monitor (Fig. 12 and ECG 4B–E)

An extrasystole is seen as an *extra* earlier QRS–T complex representing the extra ventricular contraction (and relaxation).

P wave	present.
QRS–T complex	P–R segment normal.
Heart rate	Normal, fast, slow.
	If extrasystoles are frequent, rate is irregular.
Extras	*Yes*, an extra QRS–T complex.

There is often a gap or a pause after the QRS–T of an extrasystole (ECG 5C and D). If the heart rate is fast this pause will be less obvious or absent.

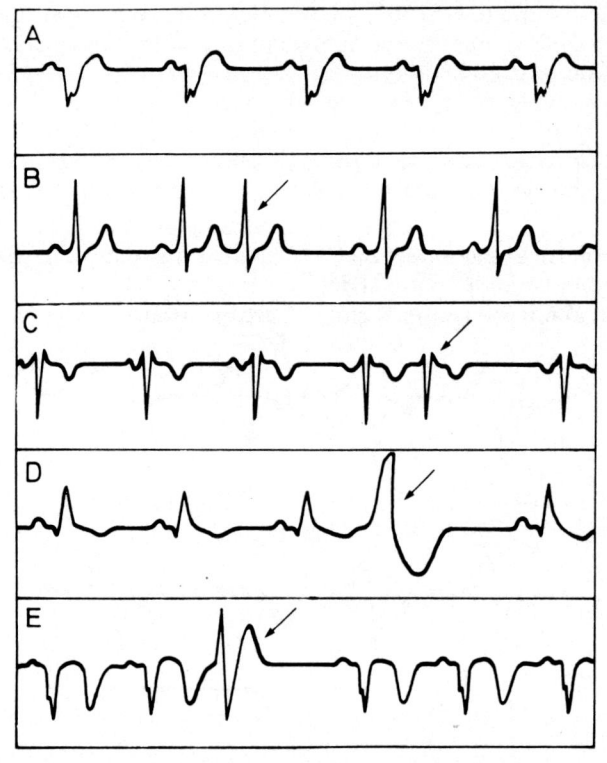

ECG 4. (A) sinus rhythm at normal heart rate; (B) and (C) atrial extrasystole; (D) and (E) ventricular extrasystole. The arrows indicate an extrasystole (an extra, earlier QRS–T complex, without a preceding P wave).

THE ARRHYTHMIAS. I   23

There are two types of extrasystoles, *atrial extrasystoles* and *ventricular extrasystoles*. The adjectives atrial and ventricular refer to whether the abnormal stimulating impulse arises in the atria or in the ventricles.

An Atrial Extrasystole (ECG 4B and C)
  1. An *extra*, usually earlier, QRS–T complex.
  2. Has *normal* configuration to QRS–T complex.
  3. Usually is *not* preceded by a P wave.

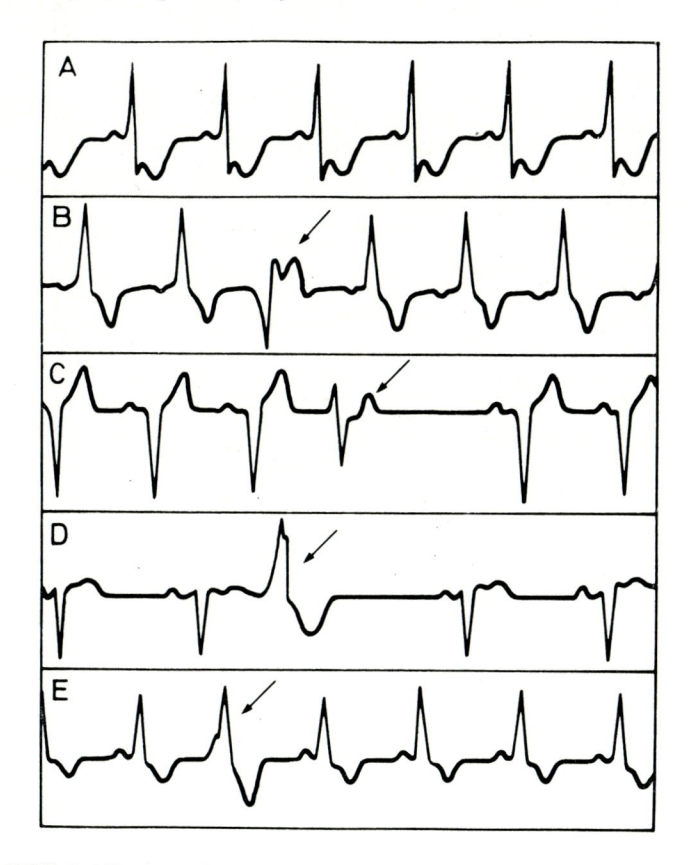

ECG 5. (A) sinus rhythm at normal heart rate; (B)–(E) ventricular extrasystoles (VES); (C) QRS–T complex of VES smaller than normal (sinus) QRS–T complex; (C) and (D) notice pause after VES; (E) less obvious VES.

A Ventricular Extrasystole (ECGs 4D and E, 5B–E and 6B–E)
  1. An *extra*, usually earlier, QRS–T complex.
  2. Has *abnormal* configuration to QRS–T complex.
  3. Is *not* preceded by a P wave.

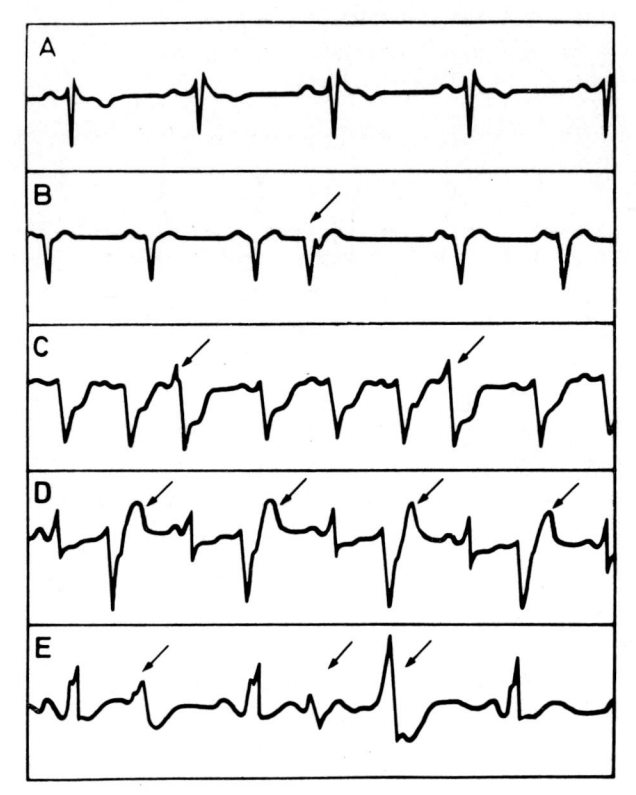

ECG 6. (A) sinus rhythm at normal heart rate; (B)–(E) ventricular extrasystole (VES); (B) less obvious VES; (C) VES falling near T wave; (D) coupling (each sinus complex followed by a VES); (E) frequent, multifocal VES.

By 'normal' or 'abnormal' configuration to QRS–T complex, is meant whether or not the configuration of the QRS–T complex of the extrasystole is identical or not to that of the normal (sinus) complexes of the trace displayed on the scope.

Thus both an atrial and a ventricular extrasystole are seen as a single extra QRS–T complex; on the scope a ventricular extrasystole never has a preceding P wave, and an atrial extrasystole usually does not have one. Sometimes with an atrial extrasystole a P wave immediately before the QRS–T complex may be recognizable.

A ventricular extrasystole is usually *easy to detect* (ECG 5D) as the configuration (i.e. size, shape and direction) of the QRS–T complex is different, often obviously so, from the normal QRS–T complexes which precede and follow it. One frequent feature of the abnormal QRS–T configuration of a ventricular extrasystole is an increase in width of the QRS complex. However, assessment from the monitor of the QRS width of QRS–T complexes is not easy.

An atrial extrasystole is less easy to spot as the extra QRS–T complex is *identical* in configuration to the normal complexes (ECG 4B and C). However, with careful monitor observation detection of an atrial extrasystole as an 'extra', earlier QRS–T complex without a preceding P wave, and followed often by a pause before the P wave of the next normal complex, is not difficult.

An atrial extrasystole has a normal configuration to the QRS–T complex because its impulse arises in the atria and is still conducted down the Bundle of His and its branches in the usual manner. The impulse of a ventricular extrasystole has a totally abnormal mode of conduction. Originating in the ventricular muscle itself it does not need to travel down the Bundle of His. It stimulates the ventricular muscle locally to contract, and then passes along the branches of the Bundle of His to stimulate the remaining ventricular muscle.

Sometimes an atrial extrasystole arises near or at the AV node when it is described as a 'nodal extrasystole'. Though this focus of origin for a nodal form of atrial extrasystole may be recognized on formal ECGs, there are no certain features to make this distinction on monitor observation.

An atrial extrasystole is also known as a 'supraventricular' extrasystole, as the abnormal impulse arises outside or 'above' the ventricles. The term atrial extrasystole is simpler and aids distinction of its origin and features from a ventricular extrasystole.

Coupling

Coupling (ECG 6D) is the term given when every (or nearly every) normal sinus complex is followed by an extrasystole, which is usually a ventricular one. A common cause of coupling is digitalis toxicity.

Significance of Extrasystoles

1. After Myocardial Infarction

Extrasystoles occur especially in the early stages of about 35 per cent of the patients with acute myocardial infarction. Atrial extrasystoles are less common and less important though they may herald the development of atrial fibrillation. However, ventricular extrasystoles following myocardial infarction are *very significant*, because they may lead on to ventricular fibrillation, i.e. cardiac arrest. Fortunately ventricular extrasystoles are the easier ones to spot.

After acute myocardial infarction, ventricular extrasystoles are particu-

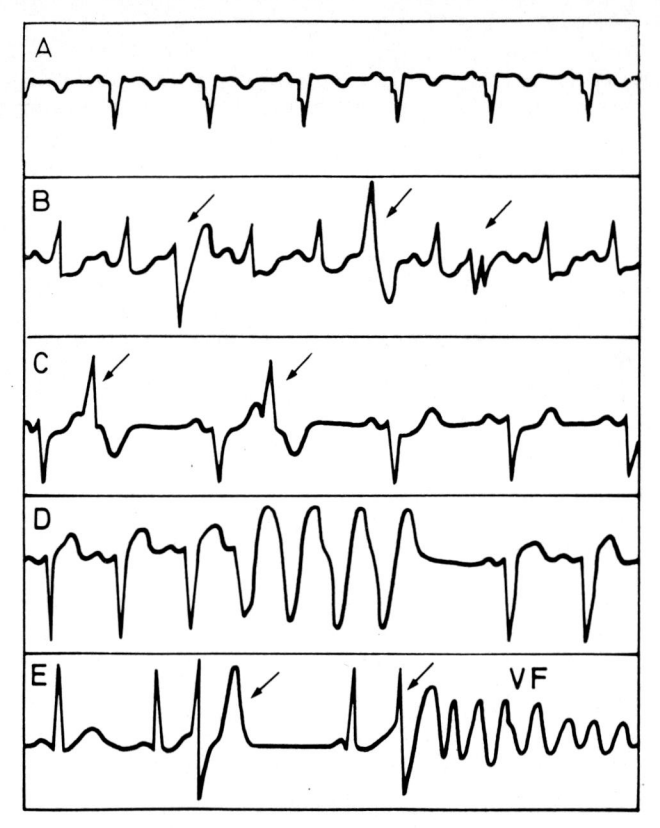

ECG 7. (A) sinus rhythm at normal heart rate; (B) frequent multifocal VES; (C) VES falling on T wave (R on T); (D) salvo of VES; (E) VES falling on T wave, leading to ventricular fibrillation (VF).

larly dangerous in their ability to precipitate either ventricular tachycardia or ventricular fibrillation when:
  (a) they are frequent, i.e. more than 6 per min;
  (b) if they fall on or near the T wave of the preceding normal QRS–T complex (ECGs 6C, 7C and E, 15B);
  (c) if their configuration is varying (ECG 7B) (because this implies their site of origin is varying, i.e. that they are 'multifocal');
  (d) if they occur in salvos (ECG 7D).

If ventricular extrasystoles have *any* of these qualities after acute myocardial infarction they should be suppressed. This is usually attempted in the first instance by intravenous lignocaine.

2. Extrasystoles with Heart Block (see p. 42)

3. Extrasystoles with Electrolyte Disturbances

A low serum potassium (hypokalaemia) may lead to extrasystoles, which are usually ventricular in type. Hypokalaemia may follow open-heart surgery or the administration of diuretics. The extrasystoles are suppressed by replacing orally or intravenously the potassium deficiency.

4. Extrasystoles and Digitalis

Extrasystoles, particularly ventricular ones in the form of coupling (ECG 6D), are a common feature of digitalis toxicity. Their appearance is an indication to reduce the dose of digitalis administered.

5. Extrasystoles at Other Times

These are less significant. They may occur in relation to age, after a heavy meal, coffee, smoking, or as a feature of many types of heart disease.

CHAPTER 5

The arrhythmias

II. Atrial and ventricular tachycardia, atrial flutter and atrial fibrillation

When atrial or ventricular extrasystoles continue without being interspersed with normal (sinus) complexes the disturbance of rhythm is called atrial or ventricular tachycardia, respectively. The impulse, instead of arising at the SA node, is continuously arising from the ectopic focus. The heart rate is fast and hence the term tachycardia is used.

On the Monitor (ECG 8B–E)

	Atrial tachycardia	*Ventricular tachycardia*
P wave	Absent (usually).	Absent.
QRS–T complex	Constant in shape. Normal width to QRS complexes.	Slight variations in shape. Tall wide QRS complexes.
Heart rate	Fast, regular.	Fast, regular.
Extras	None.	None.

As with single atrial extrasystoles, P waves sometimes may be seen in atrial tachycardia just before QRS–T complex, or sometimes just after the QRS but before the T wave.

Assessment of QRS width, of QRS–T complexes is not easy and requires experience. Sometimes the QRS may also be broader than normal in atrial tachycardia. For these reasons distinction on the monitor between atrial and ventricular tachycardia may be very difficult and a formal ECG may need to be taken. The rapid regular heart rate and absence of P waves must be spotted and alert one to the diagnosis of atrial or ventricular tachycardia.

Significance of Atrial and Ventricular Tachycardia

Both atrial and ventricular tachycardia are serious arrhythmias as the heart is made to beat too fast. Both may lead to heart failure, lower the blood pressure (hypotension) and cause cardiac chest pain (angina).

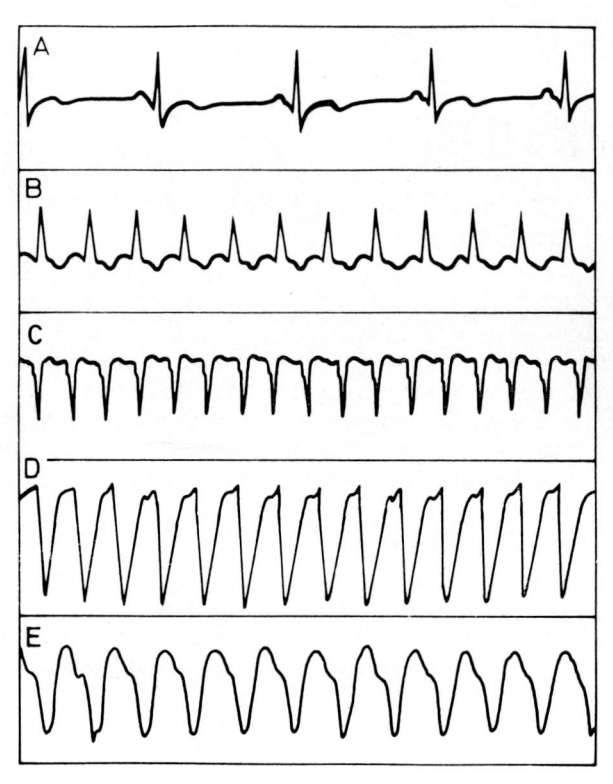

ECG 8. (A) sinus rhythm at normal heart rate; (B) and (C) atrial tachycardia; (D) and (E) ventricular tachycardia.

Ventricular tachycardia is particularly serious as it may lead to ventricular fibrillation.

Atrial tachycardia is the arrhythmia which is sometimes corrected by pressing on the neck over the division of one carotid artery, i.e. carotid sinus massage.

ATRIAL FLUTTER

This arrhythmia may be considered as a special form of atrial tachycardia, where the discharge of impulses from the ectopic atrial focus is very rapid, about 300 per min, so that the ventricles only respond and contract to some of the impulses. There are thus more atrial contractions than ventricular contractions. Each QRS–T complex is, therefore, pre-

THE ARRHYTHMIAS. II

ceded by *more than one (two to four) P wave*. There is either no gap, or at the most only a very small one, between successive P waves.

The number of extra P waves and the heart rate are dependent on the number of impulses which are able to pass down from the atria to the ventricles. In other words, both the number of extra P waves seen and the heart rate are dependent upon the number of impulses which are blocked from passing down the Bundle of His, i.e. the amount of *functional heart block*. If the block is small, e.g. 2 : 1 there will be two P waves to each QRS–T complex and the heart rate will be rapid, approximately 300 divided by 2, i.e. about 150 per min. In these cases there will be one P wave, and one extra P wave; the extra P wave is often 'buried' in or near the QRS–T complex and is then difficult to spot. The trace will thus closely resemble atrial tachycardia which, as described on p. 29 sometimes may have QRS–T complexes preceded by a P wave. A formal ECG will be necessary to distinguish whether the arrhythmia is atrial flutter or atrial tachycardia.

On the other hand, if the block is larger, e.g. 3 : 1 there will be two extra P waves between QRS–T complexes and the heart rate will be less rapid, approximately 300 divided by 3, i.e. about 100 per min. As there is more than one extra P wave, it is easier to detect that there are extra P waves present. *There is little or no gap between successive P waves* and this is an important characteristic distinguishing atrial flutter from heart block. The P waves are sometimes, but by no means always, tented in shape on the monitor trace. The absence of a gap between the extra P waves, together with their tented shape can produce a serrated appearance, the so called 'saw-tooth P waves'.

The heart rate is usually regular, but if the block is varying, the number of extra P waves will vary, and the heart rate will also be irregular.

On the Monitor (ECG 9B–E)

The trace of atrial flutter may take a number of different forms, varying between one which is fast and difficult to recognize with certainty and one which is slower and easier to recognize, if the presence of extra P waves is spotted.

P wave	Present.
QRS–T complex	Each preceded by P wave. P–R segment not prolonged. QRS–T shape—constant.
Heart rate	Fast (often), normal, but usually *not* slow. Regular (usually); irregular sometimes.

Extras   Yes—extra P waves.
No gap or only a small one, between successive P waves

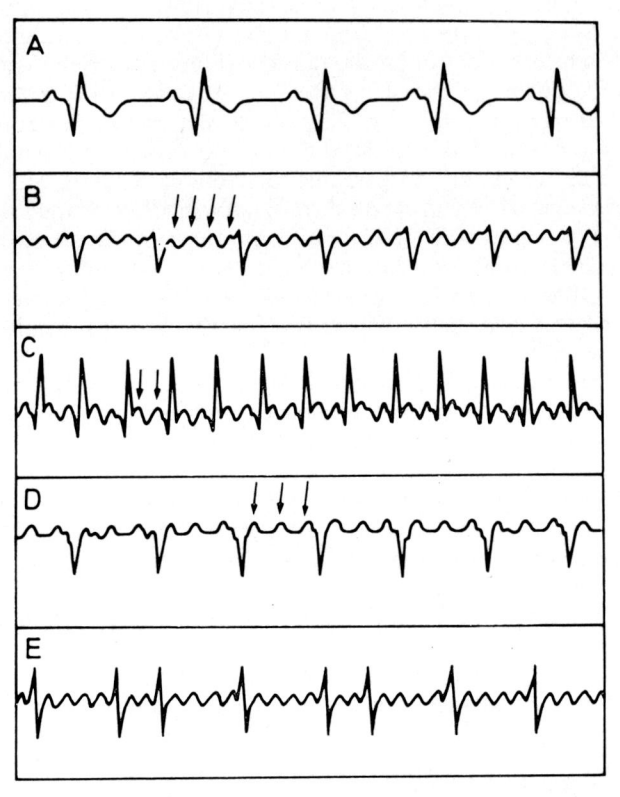

ECG 9. (A) sinus rhythm at normal heart rate; (B)–(E) atrial flutter; (B) 4 : 1 block; (C) 2 : 1 block; (D) 3 : 1 block; (E) varying block. The arrows indicate P waves.

Significance of Atrial Flutter

Atrial flutter is an uncommon arrhythmia. It may occur after myocardial infarction and heart surgery. With monitor observation its significance lies in its distinction from two other arrhythmias, *atrial tachycardia* (when the rate is fast, and distinction is often difficult) and more important still, from *heart block* (when the rate is less rapid). When the rate is fast, heart failure and hypotension may ensue.

ATRIAL FIBRILLATION (AF)

With this arrhythmia impulses no longer arise from the SA node but arise in the atria at a very rapid irregular rate of about 400 per min. The atria no longer contract but instead quiver rapidly and irregularly. There are therefore *no P waves to the ECG trace*.

Of the many impulses reaching the AV node at irregular intervals, only some are conducted down the Bundle of His to the ventricles. The ventricular contractions that occur are thus irregular in rate. *The heart rate in AF is irregular.*

On the Monitor (ECG 10B–E)

P wave	Absent.
QRS–T complex	Shape basically constant.
Heart rate	Irregular. Fast, normal or slow.
Extras	Sometimes the base-line between QRS–T complexes is irregular due to small 'fibrillation waves'.

The absence of P waves and the irregular heart rate are the diagnostic features on the monitor to identify AF.

Sometimes an impulse is conducted down the Bundle of His after a shorter period of diastole (ventricular relaxation) than usual, so that less blood will have reached the ventricles from the atria. This leads to the subsequent ventricular contraction pumping out less blood than usual. Hence a pulse beat may not always be felt at the radial artery for each ventricular contraction seen as a QRS–T complex on the scope, or heard as the heart sounds at the cardiac apex. This is the cause for the so-called 'pulse deficit' of AF, which is more marked the faster the heart rate.

The configuration of QRS–T complexes is basically constant, but just as the strength of ventricular contraction varies, so may minor variations in the height and shape of QRS–T complexes occur. They are, however, only minor variations and are not a prominent feature.

With AF the base-line between QRS–T complexes is often irregular instead of flat (ECG 10E). This is more noticeable when the heart rate is slow, as the distance between successive QRS–T complexes is larger (ECG 10C). The irregularity of the base line is due to small waves variable in number, shape and size which are associated with the quivering atria. They are known as 'fibrillation waves' and should be ignored.

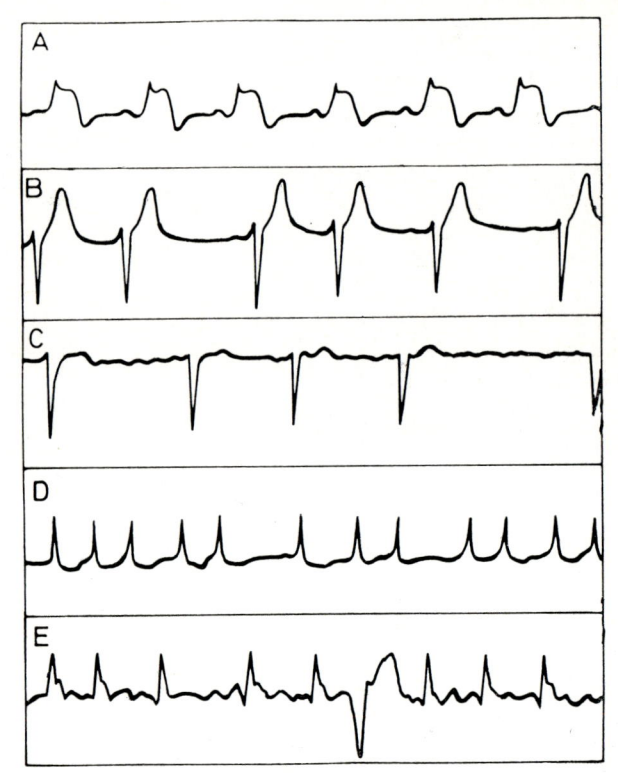

ECG 10. (A) sinus rhythm at normal heart rate; (B)–(E) atrial fibrillation (AF). Notice: (a) absence of P wave, and (b) gap between successive QRS–T complexes continuously varying. (E) AF with ventricular extrasystole.

Significance of Atrial Fibrillation

AF is common in chronic rheumatic heart disease, e.g. mitral stenosis. It may also occur after myocardial infarction, and following thoracic surgery. Sometimes it develops during pneumonia, and in thyrotoxicosis. If the heart rate is rapid, as with all tachycardias the heart will be made to beat too fast and heart failure and hypotension may ensue. The standard treatment for AF is with a digitalis preparation, e.g. digoxin, which slows the heart rate. The rhythm, however, usually persists as AF and does not revert to sinus rhythm. Of the many impulses reaching the AV node from the atria, digitalis reduces the number which cross the node to pass down the Bundle of His to reach the ventricles and so produce contraction. Digitalis is said to increase the amount of 'functional heart block'.

CHAPTER 6

The arrhythmias

III. Heart block

Heart block is an arrhythmia where there is partial or total interruption ('block') in the conduction of an impulse across the AV node and down the Bundle of His to reach the ventricles. There are three grades, called 'degrees' of heart block (HB):
 First degree.
 Second degree.
 Third degree, more commonly known as complete heart block (CHB). In all forms of heart block the heart rate is usually *slow*.

FIRST DEGREE HEART BLOCK

The passage (conduction) of an impulse across the AV node and down the Bundle of His does occur but it takes longer than usual. The P–R segment is *prolonged* as this segment represents the conduction of an impulse across the AV node and down the bundle (see p. 13).

On the Monitor (ECG 11B–C)

P wave	Present.
QRS–T complex	Each preceded by P wave.
	P–R segment—prolonged.
	QRS–T shape constant.
Heart rate	Slow, regular.
Extras	None.

Recognition on the monitor screen that the P–R segment is prolonged, is difficult.

SECOND DEGREE HEART BLOCK

There is intermittent failure of impuse conduction across the AV node and down the Bundle of His. Some of the impulses reaching the AV node do not pass down to the ventricles.
 Some P waves are, therefore, not followed by QRS–T complexes.

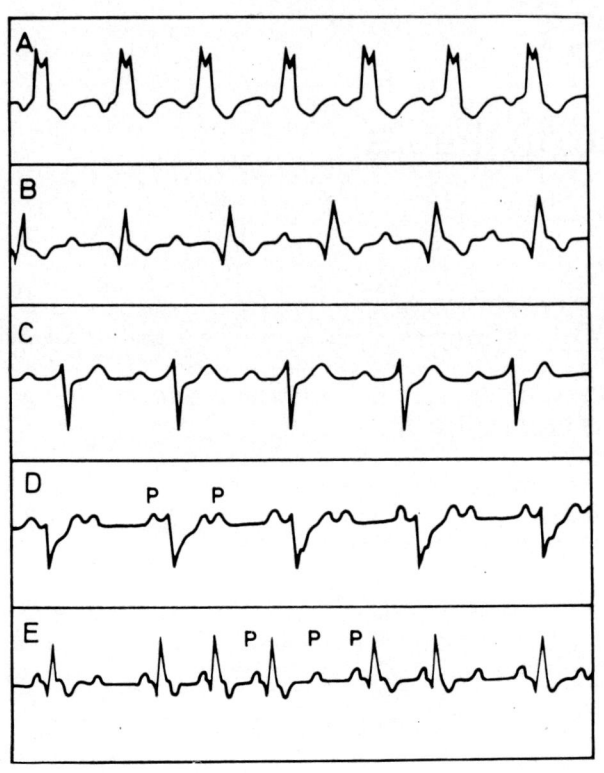

ECG 11. (A) sinus rhythm at normal heart rate; (B) and (C) first degree heart block, note length of P–R segment is constant; (D) second degree heart block; (E) second degree heart block with varying block.

On the Monitor (ECGs 11D, E and 12B)

P wave	Present.
QRS–T complex	Each preceded by P wave.
	P–R segment *constant* (and normal) in length.
	QRS–T shape constant.
Heart rate	Slow.
	Regular (usually) or irregular (sometimes).
Extras	Yes, an extra P wave after the T wave is present.
	Definite gap between successive P waves.

The failure of an impulse to be conducted across the AV node and down the Bundle of His may occur:

THE ARRHYTHMIAS. III

(a) *Regularly*, so that, for example, every second P wave is not followed by a QRS–T complex. On the monitor screen (ECGs 11D and 12B) an apparent extra P wave after each T wave will be seen, which must not be confused for a U wave. The QRS–T complexes occur regularly, i.e. the heart rate is slow, but regular.

(b) *Irregularly*, when every now and then a P wave is not followed by a QRS–T complex, i.e. the QRS–T complex is absent or 'dropped' (ECG 11E). As the QRS–T complex is 'dropped' irregularly, the heart rate is irregular. *Note:* unlike the Wenckebach phenomenon (see below) there is no progressive lengthening of the P–R segment before a QRS–T complex is 'dropped'.

The heart rate is judged by an assessment of the distance between the spikes of successive QRS–T complexes.

WENCKEBACH PHENOMENON

This phenomenon is a form of heart block intermediate between first degree and second degree heart block. There is a progressive increase in duration of conduction of an impulse across the AV node and down the Bundle of His, until one impulse is not conducted so that a ventricular contraction does not occur. The process is then repeated.

On the Monitor (ECG 12C and D)

P wave	Present.
QRS–T complex	*P–R segment*—progressive lengthening with successive complexes until a QRS–T is 'dropped', i.e. a P wave is not followed by a QRS–T. Process is then repeated.
Heart rate	Slow. Irregular, due to dropped beats.
Extras	None.

Usually it is the third to fifth QRS–T complex of the sequence which is dropped. On the scope, the Wenckebach phenomenon is easy to recognize.

COMPLETE HEART BLOCK (CHB)

There is total block at the AV node or along the Bundle of His so that no impulse may pass down the Bundle to the ventricles. However, the ventricles still contract, as a ventricular pacemaker starts up somewhere in the ventricular muscle. The rate of ventricular contraction (and therefore of QRS–T complexes, and the pulse) is *slow*, about 30 to 50 per min, but *regular*. The atrial contraction rate (and therefore of P waves) is

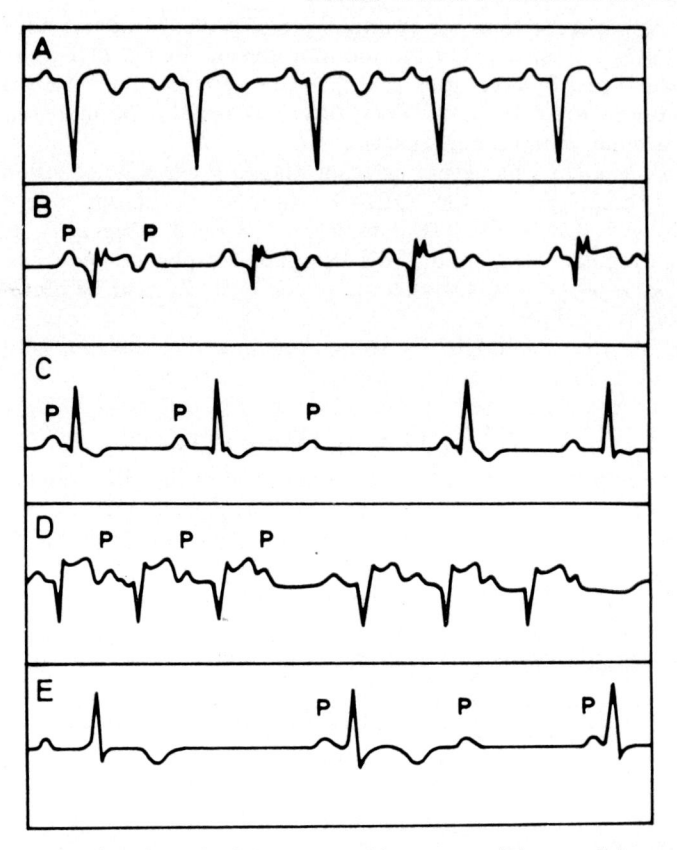

ECG 12. (A) sinus rhythm at normal heart rate; (B) second degree heart block; (C) and (D) Wenckebach phenomenon, progressive lengthening of P–R segment until a QRS–T complex is dropped; (E) complete heart block.

normal, about 70 per min. Hence there are more atrial contractions than ventricular contractions, i.e. *more P waves than QRS–T complexes*. As the atria and ventricles are stimulated by different pacemakers they beat completely independently of each other, i.e. *P waves and QRS–T complexes bear no relationship in their timing*.

These features are manifested by the *distance between P waves and QRS–T complexes continuously varying* sometimes small, sometimes large. Hence the apparent P–R segment is continuously varying in length. Unlike the Wenckebach phenomenon, there is no progressive increase in

THE ARRHYTHMIAS. III

the length of the P–R segment, no dropped QRS–T complexes, and the heart rate is regular. The continuously varying 'apparent P–R segment' is the diagnostic feature of CHB with monitor observation.

On the Monitor (ECG 12E and 13B–E)

P wave	Present.
QRS–T complex	*P–R segment continuously varying in length.*
	QRS–T shape may be large and wide, and may vary slightly.
Heart rate	Slow.
	Regular.
Extras	Yes, extra P waves.

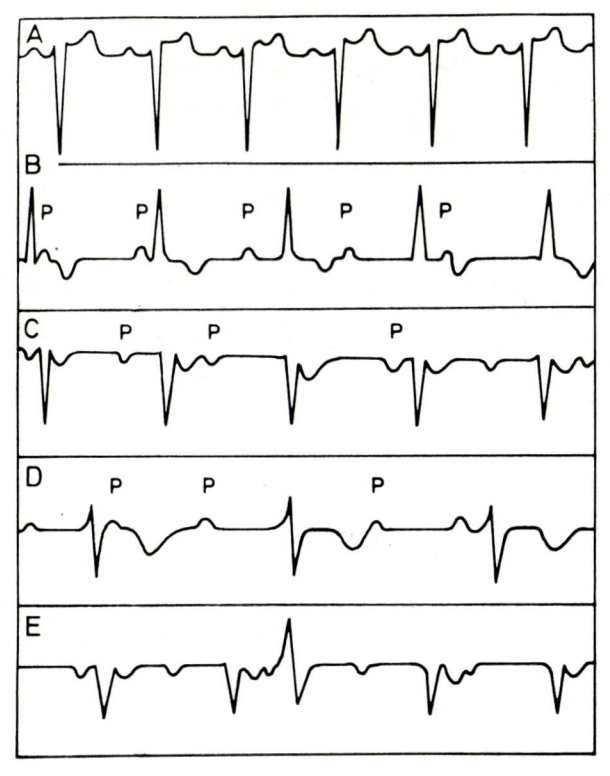

ECG 13. (A) sinus rhythm at normal heart rate; (B)–(E) complete heart block (CHB); (E) CHB with a ventricular extrasystole. Note 'apparent P–R segment' in CHB continuously varies in length.

Notice, that the term 'apparent P–R segment' is used. In CHB as no conduction of impulses down the Bundle of His occurs, the atria and ventricles beat independently. As the P–R segment represents impulse conduction across the AV node and down the Bundle (see p. 13) there can be no true P–R segment. However, as P waves and QRS–T complexes are occurring on the same trace, there must be a gap between the QRS–T complex and the last P wave preceding it, i.e. the 'apparent P–R segment'.

As P waves and QRS–T complexes occur independently, and as the P wave rate is faster than that of the QRS–T complexes, the P waves may be considered to 'walk through the QRS–T complexes'. Indeed, a P wave may sometimes be clearly seen as a little 'bump' actually on a QRS–T complex (ECG 13D). The QRS–T complexes may, therefore, vary a little in shape.

Recognition of Heart Block

Heart block is difficult to appreciate from the monitor. In first degree heart block, the trace looks normal. In second degree heart block and CHB, though there are extra P waves they are not numerous, and are often difficult to spot unless the trace is specifically observed for extra P waves.

The feature to draw one's attention to the possibility of heart block is a *slow heart rate*; whenever the heart rate is 60 or less, be particularly on the look out for heart block.

In first degree heart block, the trace looks normal (ECG 11B and C) since to spot that the P–R segment is prolonged is particularly difficult, and only after considerable experience at monitor observation will this difference be appreciated. On the other hand, the progressive lengthening over successive complexes of the P–R segment, culminating in a 'dropped' QRS–T complex, makes the Wenckebach phenomenon easy to recognize (ECG 14E).

In second degree and complete heart block the trace shows extra P waves between QRS–T complexes but these may be difficult to detect as they are not numerous. However, the continuously varying 'apparent P–R segment' of CHB (ECG 12E) is not difficult to appreciate if the monitor trace is carefully observed. In second degree heart block, the heart rate may be regular or irregular, but with CHB it is *always* regular.

Distinction between Atrial Flutter and Second Degree Heart Block or CHB

It will be remembered that in atrial flutter (see p. 30), extra P waves between QRS–T complexes also occur. This is because there is a rapid

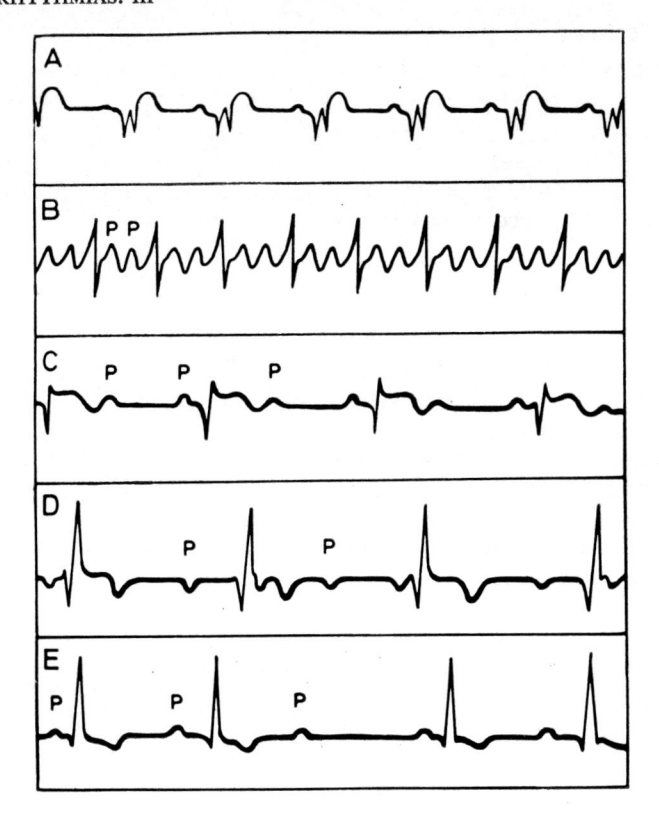

ECG 14. (A) sinus rhythm at normal heart rate; (B) atrial flutter; (C) second degree heart block; (D) complete heart block; (E) Wenckebach phenomenon. Notice no gap between P waves with atrial flutter, and the clear gap between P waves in heart block.

discharge of impulses (about 300 per min) from an ectopic atrial pacemaker, and not all the impulses are conducted across the AV node and down the Bundle of His, i.e. there is functional heart block. However, the rate of the P waves (300 per min) is very rapid, so that there is no clear gap, or only a very small one, between successive P waves (ECG 14B). In second degree heart block and CHB the atrial rate and hence that of the P waves, is normal say about 70 per min. There is a clear return to the flat base line at the end of each P wave, i.e. a clear gap between successive P waves (ECG 14C and D).

On the Monitor (ECG 14B–D)
The distinguishing features are:

	Atrial flutter	*Second degree and CHB*
Heart rate	Rapid (100 or more per min)	Slow (60 or less per min)
P waves	Little or no gap between successive P waves	Clear gap between successive P waves

Complete Heart Block and Extrasystoles

Just as when the heart rate is *slow*, one should be on the look out for heart block, so when the rhythm is known to be CHB the trace should be carefully watched for ventricular extrasystoles (ECGs 13E and 16C). They may occur spontaneously or be precipitated by treatment, e.g. with isoprenaline. When ventricular extrasystoles occur with CHB there is a risk of ventricular tachycardia or ventricular fibrillation. The usual features of a ventricular extrasystole will generally apply, i.e. an extra, earlier QRS–T complex of different configuration to the normal QRS–T complexes.

Significance of Heart Block

Just as a heart rate which is too fast impairs the pumping action of diseased heart muscle, so a heart rate which is too slow, as may occur in CHB, may lead to heart failure, breathlessness and hypotension.

In CHB recurrent short episodes of cardiac arrest, which usually revert back to CHB spontaneously, may occur. In these episodes, called *Stokes–Adams* attacks, cardiac asystole or rapid ventricular tachycardia lead to the patient loosing consciousness, becoming pulseless with dilated pupils. The arrest usually ceases spontaneously, or after treatment consisting of a sharp, firm thud over the sternum with a closed first. There is always the risk however, that even after the full treatment for cardiac arrest, the heart may not restart beating effectively.

Heart block (all degrees) may be:

(1) *Temporary*—after myocardial infarction; with certain fevers, e.g. acute rheumatic fever, diphtheria; or due to digitalis toxicity.

(2) *Permanent*—usually in the form of CHB in elderly patients; or rarely after cardiac surgery.

CHB and occasionally second degree heart block may be treated by cardiac pacing to speed up the heart rate to normal (see p. 45). Alternatively medical treatment with isoprenaline or atropine may be tried. In first and second degree heart block usually no specific therapy is necessary.

CHAPTER 7

Cardiac arrest

Cardiac arrest is the condition where the heart stops beating effectively. The patient loses consciousness, becomes pulseless (feel for the big arteries, e.g. carotids or femorals) and the pupils dilate.

Cardiac arrest should be diagnosed by observation of the patient, and the monitor used to show the type of rhythm disturbance.

The two arrhythmias causing cardiac arrest are:
   (1) Ventricular fibrillation (VF).
   (2) Cardiac asystole.

Ventricular Fibrillation

The ventricles cease to contract and instead quiver rapidly and ineffectively.

On the Monitor (ECG 15B–D)

A rapid irregular wavy line of large or small height (coarse or fine VF) is seen.

Occasionally cardiac arrest may be due to rapid ventricular tachycardia (VT) and sometimes the trace may be intermediate between VT and VF (sometimes referred to as 'ventricular flutter').

Cardiac Asystole

The ventricles are still.

On the Monitor (ECG 15E)

Only a flat line is seen, no complexes or waves at all being present.

Initial treatment of cardiac arrest is by external cardiac massage and by mouth-to-mouth artificial respiration. VF (and VT) may be corrected by applying an electric shock across the chest—'defibrillation'. Cardiac pacing may be attempted for cardiac asystole. During cardiac arrest sodium bicarbonate to correct acidosis, and other drugs may be administered intravenously. Resuscitation is more often successful from VF than cardiac asystole.

An important aim of cardiac monitoring is to detect less serious arrhythmias which might precipitate a cardiac arrest. By treating a less

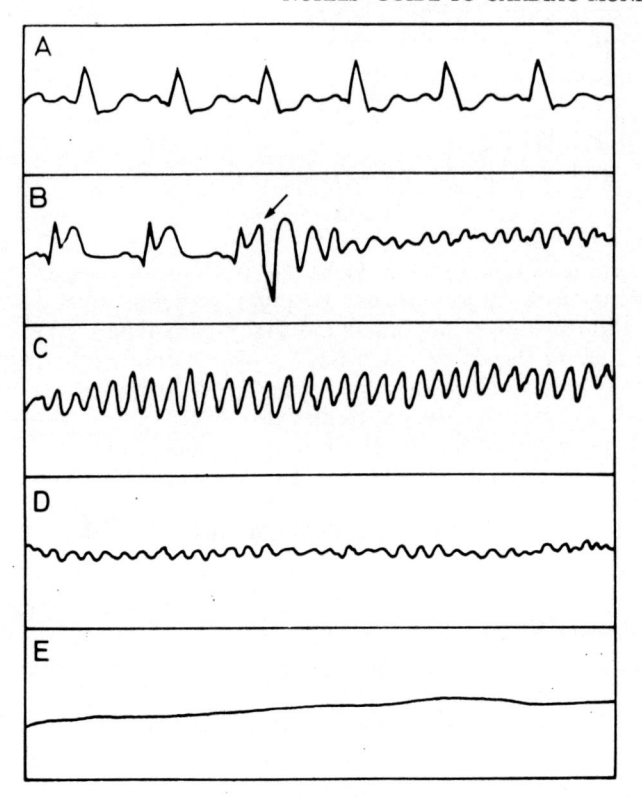

ECG 15. (A) sinus rhythm at normal heart rate; (B), (C) and (D) ventricular fibrillation (VF); (E) cardiac asystole; (B) ventricular extrasystole (arrow) falling on T wave ('R on T') precipitating VF; (C) coarse VF; (D) fine VF.

serious arrhythmia, a more grave one may be avoided later. Suppression of ventricular extrasystoles after acute myocardial infarction (p. 26) may prevent the development of VT or VF. Similarly, with complete heart block (p. 42), by increasing the heart rate for example by cardiac pacing, the risk of cardiac arrest from cardiac asystole, VF, or VT may be reduced.

Cardiac arrest is a medical emergency of the utmost urgency. All nurses must be thoroughly versed in its management and the procedures to be adopted when it occurs. This includes knowledge of the hospital telephone number to be dialled to summon aid. For a more detailed description of the management and treatment of cardiac arrest, standard textbooks should be consulted.

CHAPTER 8

Cardiac pacing

Cardiac pacing is a method to stimulate the ventricles to contract regularly by supplying electrical impulses to them. Cardiac pacing is performed for:
 1. Complete heart block (CHB) and rarely second degree heart block, to speed up the slow heart rate.
 2. Less commonly for cardiac asystole, to produce ventricular contractions. In this emergency situation, pacing may be done by supplying regular electrical shocks across the chest wall.

The slow heart rate of CHB as explained on p. 42 may lead to breathlessness, heart failure, hypotension and Stokes–Adams attacks. The heart rate may be increased by intravenous atropine, or intravenous/oral isoprenaline; the latter drug may produce ventricular extrasystoles with the consequent risk of ventricular tachycardia or ventricular fibrillation. Often, therefore, cardiac pacing is instituted.

An insulated wire with an uncovered smooth tip, called a *'catheter electrode'* is introduced into an arm or neck vein, and passed under X-ray screening to the cavity of the right ventricle, where the tip is wedged against the wall of the cavity (see Figs 13 and 14). A battery powered unit, called a *pacemaker*, which discharges an electrical impulse 70 to 80 times per min is connected to the catheter electrode. There may be another wire, called the *indifferent or skin electrode* passing from the pacemaker onto or beneath the skin, which completes the circuit. The heart is now stimulated to contract at the normal rate by impulses supplied by the pacemaker. Each QRS–T complex, instead of being preceded by a P wave, is now preceded by an impulse from the pacemaker, termed the *pacing impulse*. This is seen as a narrow bright vertical line *immediately* before each QRS–T complex (Fig. 15). The size of the pacing impulse may be large or small, and a channel on the monitor should be selected which shows it clearly. The QRS–T complexes with pacing, are often very large and wide, but they should be constant in shape. Sometimes P waves may be seen between and on QRS–T complexes; they may be ignored as the pacing impulse is now given the attention previously devoted to the P waves. P waves falling occasionally on a QRS–T complex may produce slight variations in shape to these complexes.

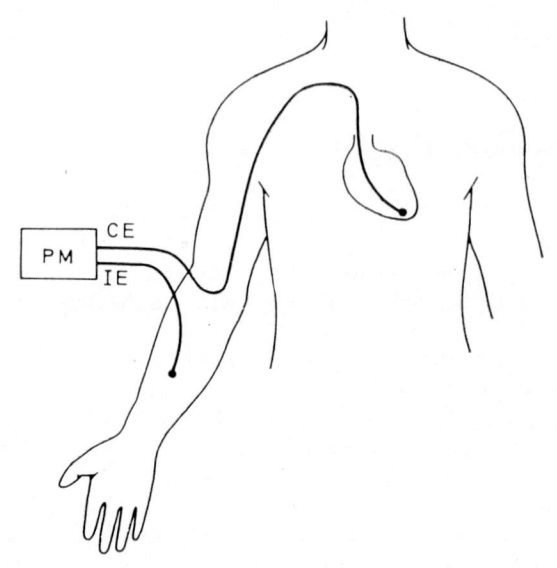

FIG. 13. Cardiac pacing. PM, pacemaker; CE, catheter electrode; IE, indifferent electrode.

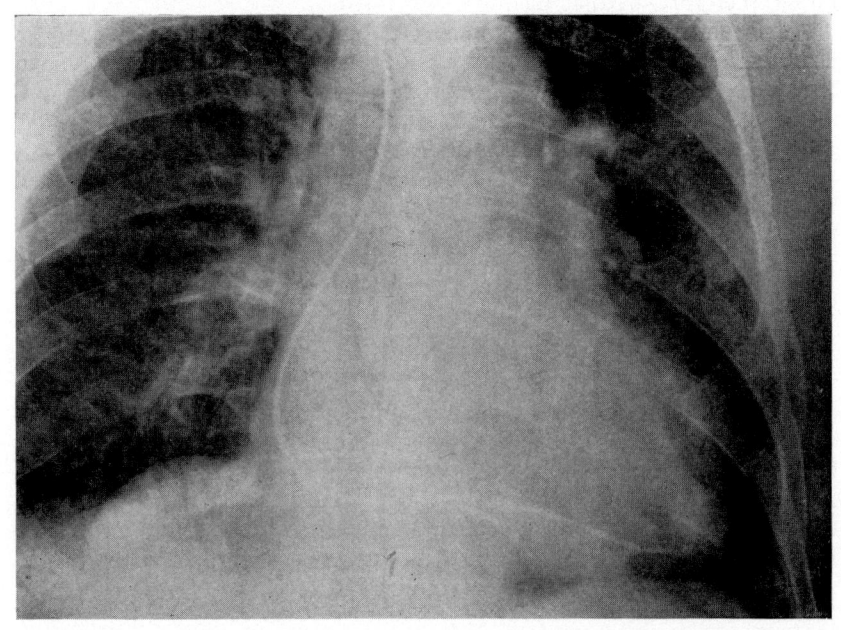

FIG. 14. X-ray showing position of catheter electrode in the heart.

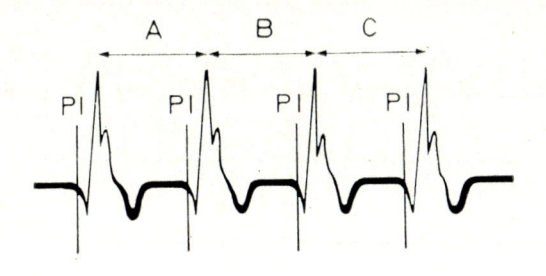

CARDIAC PACING 47

Fig. 15. Pacing impulse (PI) can be seen as a narrow bright vertical line immediately before each QRS–T complex.

On the Monitor

The trace should be observed frequently, sufficiently, and carefully to ensure that pacing is satisfactory. Careful observation is achieved in the usual manner, except that the pacing impulse has replaced the P wave. Hence observe the monitor carefully (ECGs 16D, 17A, 18A and 19A) for:

Pacing impulse	Present/absent.
QRS–T complex	Ensure each is *immediately* preceded by a pacing impulse.
	QRS–T shape constant.
Heart rate	At correct rate.
	Regular.
Extras	Are there extra pacing impulses or QRS–T complexes present?

Note that each QRS–T complex should be immediately preceded by a pacing impulse. There should be no gap between the pacing impulse and the QRS–T, equivalent to the P–R segment.

THREE DISTURBANCES OF PACING

1. Loss of Pacing Impulse

No pacing impulse is present. Pacing is, therefore, not occurring and the rhythm is again CHB, i.e. *slow* (ECG 16B).

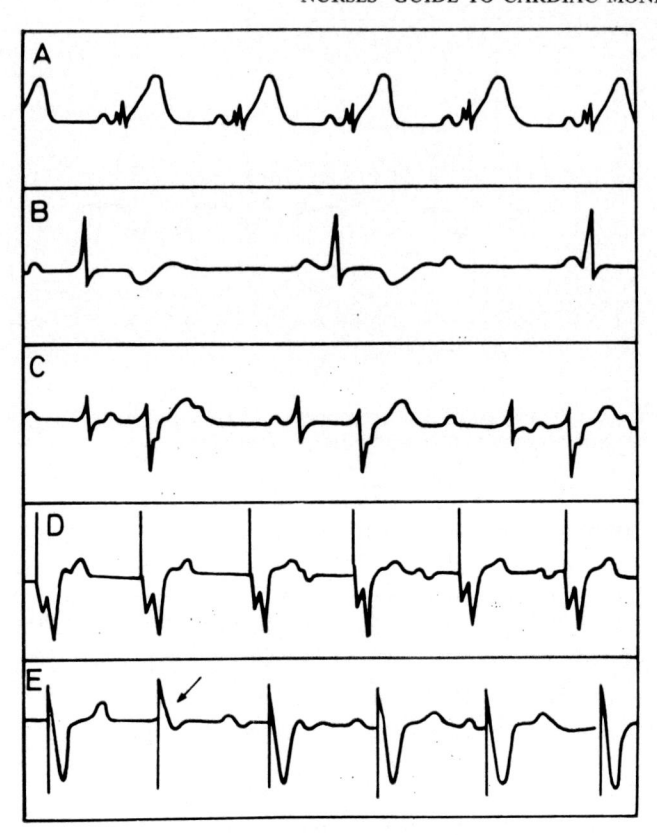

ECG 16. (A) sinus rhythm at normal heart rate; (B) complete heart block (CHB); (C) CHB with extrasystoles; (D) normal pacing; (E) weak pacing impulse (PI). The arrow indicates PI not followed by QRS–T.

On the Monitor (ECG 16B)

Pacing impulse	Absent.
QRS–T complex	Present, constant in shape.
Heart rate	*Slow*. Regular.
Extras	None.

As a first measure, check that the pacemaker is switched on, and that the connections between it and the catheter plus indifferent electrodes are not loose. Ensure that indifferent electrode has not become displaced from the skin. If the catheter and indifferent electrodes have become

CARDIAC PACING

disconnected from the pacemaker, the skin (indifferent) electrode which is the positive one, is connected to the red terminal on the pacemaker. These facts can be remembered by the eponym—RIPS—red, indifferent, positive, skin.

2. Weak Pacing Impulse

The pacing impulses are intermittently or continuously of insufficient strength to produce a ventricular contraction. Hence pacing impulses are *present*, but intermittently or continuously they are not followed immediately by QRS–T complexes. There are three grades of weak pacing impulse: (a) occasional single weak pacing impulse, (b) continuous weak pacing impulse, and (c) intermediate grade weak pacing impulse.

Occasional Single Weak Pacing Impulse

Occasionally one pacing impulse is not immediately followed by a QRS–T complex, i.e. one QRS–T complex is absent or 'dropped'. The next pacing impulse is immediately followed by a QRS–T complex.

On the Monitor (ECGs 16E and 17B)

Pacing impulse	Present.
QRS–T complex	Occasionally one is missing or 'dropped'.
Heart rate	Nearly at correct rate of pacemaker: irregular due to dropped beats.
Extras	None.

Continuous Weak Pacing Impulse

This is the severest grade of weak pacing impulse. Pacing impulses are present but *none* produce ventricular contraction. The cardiac rhythm is therefore the one that was present before pacing was started, i.e. complete heart block, which is *slow* and *regular*. Pacing impulses and QRS–T complexes now occur independently, i.e. pacing impulses are not immediately followed by QRS–T complexes, and QRS–T complexes are not continuously preceded immediately by pacing impulses. As the rate of pacing impulses is faster than that of the QRS–T complexes, apparent 'extra' pacing impulses will be seen between QRS–T complexes, and the gap between a pacing impulse and the next QRS–T complex will be continuously varying. Occasionally a pacing impulse will fall on a QRS–T complex and distort its shape.

On the Monitor (ECG 18B and C)

Pacing impulse	Present; not immediately followed by QRS–T complex.
QRS–T complex	Not preceded immediately by pacing impulse. Gap between pacing impulse and QRS–T complex continuously varying. QRS–T shape constant (except when a pacing impulse falls on a QRS–T complex).
Heart rate	*Slow*, regular.
Extras	Apparent extra pacing impulses.

Intermediate Grade of Weak Pacing Impulse

This form of weak pacing impulse is intermediate between the other two grades. Some pacing impulses do produce a ventricular contraction, and others do not. Some ventricular contractions are produced by the pacemaker, and some arise spontaneously. Hence in this grade:

1. Pacing impulses are present.
2. QRS–T complexes are of two types: (i) paced—immediately preceded by pacing impulse; and (ii) non-paced—not immediately preceded by pacing impulse. Usually the configuration of the two types of QRS–T complexes is different.

On the Monitor (ECG 17C–E)

Pacing impulse	Present, often not immediately followed by QRS–T complex.
QRS–T complex	Two types (paced and non-paced) with different configurations.
Heart rate	*Irregular*, slower than correct rate of pacemaker.
Extras	Apparent extra pacing impulses and QRS–T complexes.

Thus the pacing disturbance of a weak pacing impulse can produce a variable picture on the monitor, but all grades of the disturbance are easy to spot. With an occasional single weak pacing impulse, a 'dropped' QRS–T complex is easy to appreciate. Similarly, with a continuous weak pacing impulse, the slow heart-rate with constant QRS–T shape and a gap between a pacing impulse and the succeeding QRS–T complex which is continuously varying in length, are not difficult features to recognize. The irregular bizarre pattern of the intermediate grade with two types of QRS–T complexes points to an obvious disorder of pacing. Occasionally

CARDIAC PACING 51

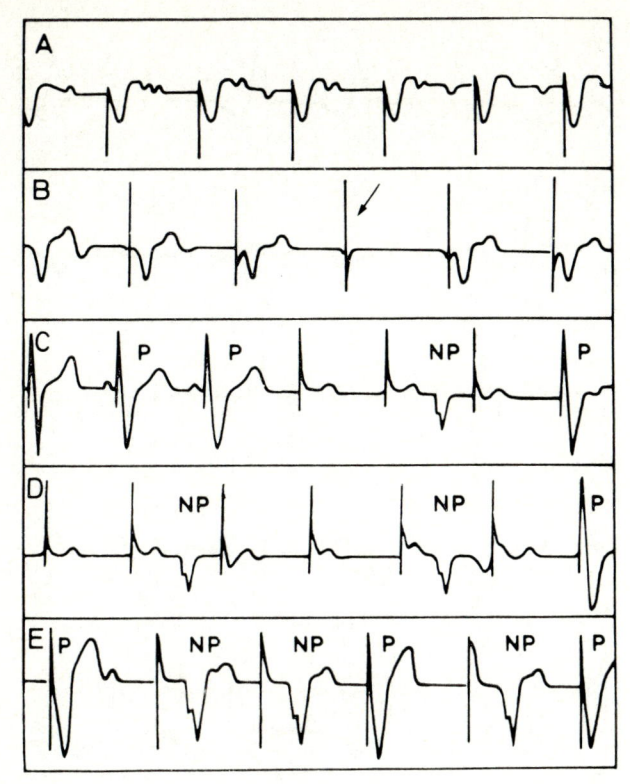

ECG 17. (A) normal pacing; (B) occasional weak pacing impulse (PI); (C)–(E) intermediate grade of weak PI. Notice QRS–T complexes of two types: paced (P) and non-paced (NP).

distinction between this last pacing disturbance and the presence of extrasystoles may be difficult.

Weak pacing impulse is corrected by increasing the strength of the pacing impulse, and/or, by repositioning the tip of the catheter electrode in the right ventricle

3. Ventricular Extrasystoles (Competition)

Pacing is satisfactory but ventricular extrasystoles occur, and are said to 'compete' with the pacemaker, as they too may produce ventricular contraction. They have the usual features of a ventricular extrasystole, i.e. an extra, earlier QRS–T complex of different configuration to the paced QRS–T complexes, and are not immediately preceded by a pacing

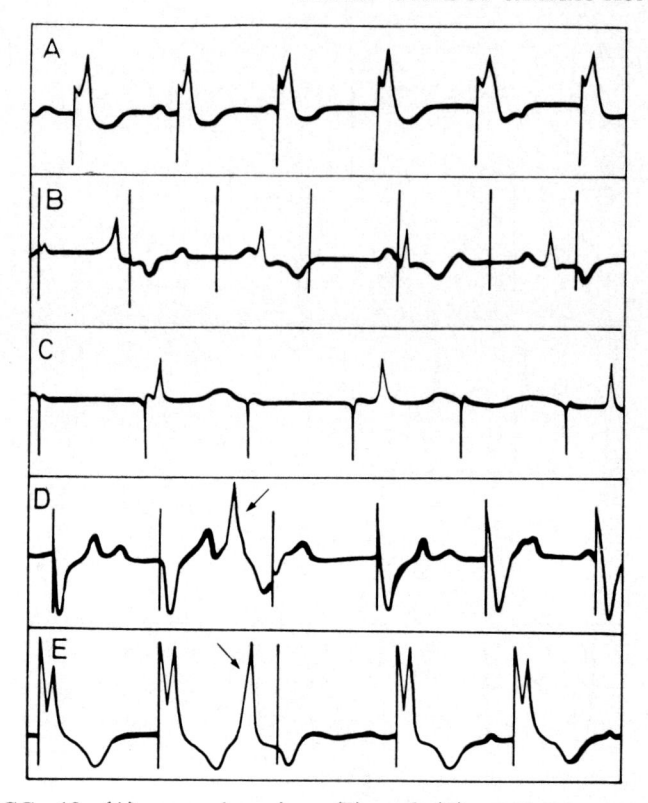

ECG. 18. (A) normal pacing; (B) and (C) continuous weak pacing impulse (PI), PI and QRS–T complexes occur independently; (D) and (E) competition-pacing disturbed by extrasystole (arrow).

impulse (ECGs 18D, E and 19B). There may be a pause after the extrasystole in which the pacing impulse will fall but will not be followed by a QRS–T complex. Competition, i.e. the presence of extrasystoles, may be corrected by increasing the pacing rate (the rate at which impulses are delivered) or by changing the position of the catheter electrode tip. Sometimes drugs may be prescribed to suppress ventricular extrasystoles.

Sinus Rhythm and Pacing

In CHB following acute myocardial infarction, the block is nearly always temporary, and sinus rhythm returns after a few days. Pacing is

CARDIAC PACING 53

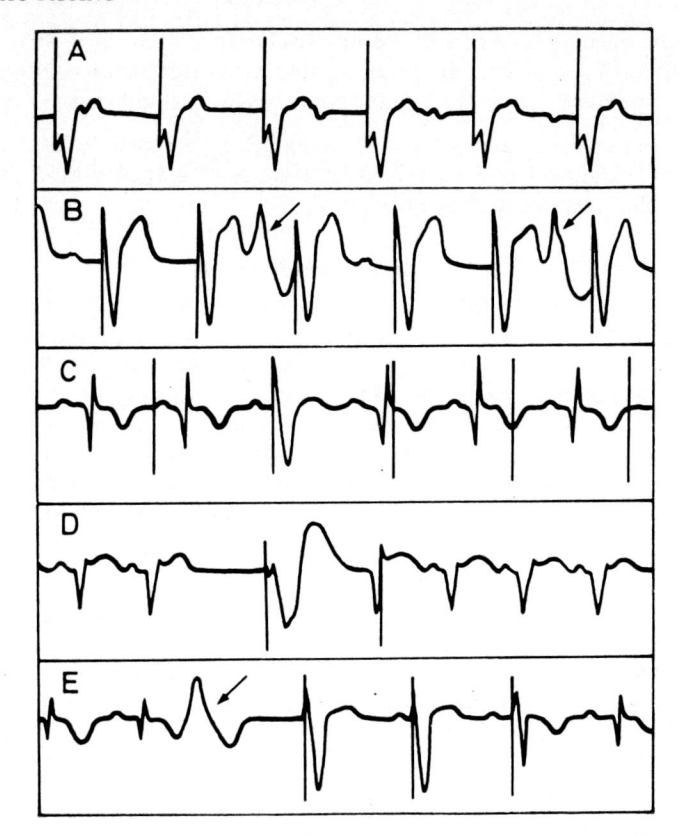

ECG 19. (A) normal pacing; (B) competition (the arrows indicate extrasystoles); (C) pacing and sinus rhythm; (D) and (E) demand pacing—pacing impulse is supplied when gap after a QRS–T complex is too long.

then no longer necessary. It is important to recognize when sinus rhythm returns (ECG 19C), and then to stop pacing as otherwise a pacing impulse may fall on a T wave, and like a ventricular extrasystole perhaps precipitate ventricular tachycardia or ventricular fibrillation.

On the Monitor (ECG 19C)
1. Sinus rhythm   Most QRS–T complexes preceded by a P wave.
2. Pacing impulses Most not followed immediately by a QRS–T complex.

3. Some paced QRS–T complexes immediately preceded by a pacing impulse, and have a different configuration to the non-paced QRS–T complexes.

This problem of a pacemaker supplying pacing impulses when they are no longer required has been solved by the use of a special type of pacemaker, called the *demand pacemaker*.

Demand Pacemaker

This type of pacemaker is becoming more frequently used. The pacemaker previously described, supplied pacing impulses to stimulate the ventricles, at a fixed or constant rate. A demand pacemaker only supplies pacing impulses when they are needed, i.e. if the heart rate is too slow. If the distance (i.e. time interval) between two QRS–T complexes is too great then a pacing impulse is supplied to produce a ventricular contraction and so increase the heart rate. If the heart rate is faster than the rate set on the demand pacemaker, then no pacing impulses are supplied.

On the Monitor (ECG 19D and E)

QRS–T complexes: When the gap after one QRS–T becomes too long a pacing impulse followed immediately by a paced QRS–T complex occurs. Pacing impulses with paced QRS–T complexes continue until heart takes over, when non-paced QRS–T complexes will reappear and pacing impulses will disappear.

Usually non-paced, and paced QRS–T complexes have a different configuration which aids their distinction.

Sometimes the gap after a QRS–T complex is too long because an extrasystole has occurred—the excessive gap representing the pause which often follows an extrasystole. During this pause a pacing impulse will be supplied by the pacemaker (ECG 19E).

When sinus rhythm returns after CHB with acute myocardial infarction, as the sinus rhythm rate is faster (i.e. normal) pacing impulses will no longer be supplied by the demand pacemaker.

Monitor observation of patients with pacemakers has been given in some detail as it is important to discover whether pacing is no longer satisfactory. If this chapter has been difficult to understand, wait until caring for a patient with a pacemaker and then study the monitor trace, being on the look out for the three disturbances described (i.e. loss of the pacing impulse, a weak pacing impulse or competition).

CHAPTER 9

General notes and hints on monitor observation

1. Observe the Monitor

This must be done frequently, sufficiently and carefully (see p. 15). The more often the monitor is observed the sooner one will become accustomed to the normal trace and be able to recognize arrhythmias.

Whenever practical, never walk past a monitor without observing the trace.

2. The Patient Comes First

Remember the patient is more important than the monitor! Never neglect patient observation for that of the monitor.

3. Doubts

If there is any doubt whether the trace is normal or has changed, inform staff nurse, sister or the houseman.

4. Rhythm not Shape

Monitoring is performed to confirm that the heart's rhythm of contraction is normal or to detect that it is abnormal (an arrhythmia). The shape, size and direction (the configuration) of the waves is much less important. Similarly, whether there is elevation or depression of the S–T segment is not important with monitoring observation.

5. Flat Line on the Scope

Though this may be due to cardiac asystole (see p. 43) look first at the patient. If he is obviously alright and fully conscious cardiac arrest has not occurred and cardiac asystole is not the cause of the flat trace. Check the connections: the patient cable may have come out of its socket on the monitor; the leads may not be connected to the electrodes, and rarely all the electrodes may have become displaced. Some monitors have a channel, marked 'O', which only displays a flat-line. If the knob controlling the size of the trace (sometimes called 'gain') has been turned fully down, then the trace may also only show a flat line.

6. The 'Fuzzy' Trace—Interference Pattern

Sometimes after applying the electrodes, particularly chest electrodes, to the skin, the trace instead of being a thin line, is a 'fuzzy' broad line (ECGs 20B and 1A). Also a trace initially satisfactory, may later develop

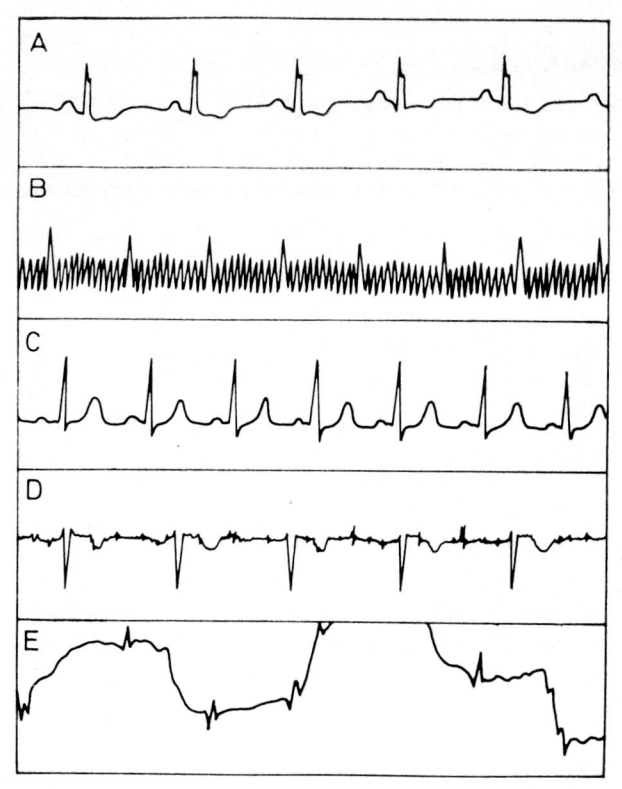

ECG 20. (A) sinus rhythm at normal heart rate; (B) the 'fuzzy' trace; (C) trace of (B) corrected; (D) the 'spikey' trace; (E) wandering base-line.

this characteristic, which obscures the P and T waves. To obtain a thin clear trace carry out *in sequence* the following manoeuvres until the 'fuzzy' trace is corrected:

(a) Adjust focus on the monitor.
(b) Alter channel on the monitor.
(c) Look for and remove any source of electricity near the bed, e.g. mains cable of the monitor or an electric light on or over the bed, or a patient 'buzzer' on the bed. These sources must be removed or taken as far away from the bed as possible.
(d) Remove and reinsert the plug of the mains cable into the same or another mains socket.
(e) Change leads of patient cable from one electrode to another.
(f) Replace electrodes, one at a time, *thoroughly cleaning the skin* before reapplying the electrode.

Hence, if the trace is 'fuzzy', do not immediately pull off all the electrodes; instead check whether the trace may be corrected by a simpler remedy. Rarely, if all these measures have been unsuccessful, or it the problem is a recurrent one, seek the advice of the senior ECG technician. As this problem is within his field of interest he should be pleased to give assistance. Sometimes an 'earthing wire' that is, a wire with a bull-dog clip at either end which is connected from a metal part of the bed (e.g. a part scraped free of paint) to a nearby pipe/radiator or a metal screw on the monitor, will 'cure' the monitor trace of interference.

In an emergency where immediate monitoring is required, if a 'fuzzy' trace is obtained with chest electrodes there may not be time to carry out the corrective manoeuvres. In this situation it is better to apply limb electrodes, as they are less susceptible to this disturbance, which is also known as 'A–C interference'.

7. The 'Spikey' Trace (ECG 20D)

Unlike the uniform fuzziness of the previous trace, this trace is occasionally and irregularly interrupted by spikes of varying height. It is due to muscle movements. Ask the patient to lie still and relax, and it will disappear.

8. The Wandering Base-Line (ECG 20E)

Instead of a trace which crosses the screen at the same level, the trace wanders up and down, particularly with deep respiratory movements. This trace is due to faulty electrode(s) which should be replaced.

9. Extras (ECG 21B–E)

Always be on the look out for extra waves or QRS–T complexes on the trace. These may either be large and spikey—an extra QRS–T complex, i.e. an extrasystole which may be:

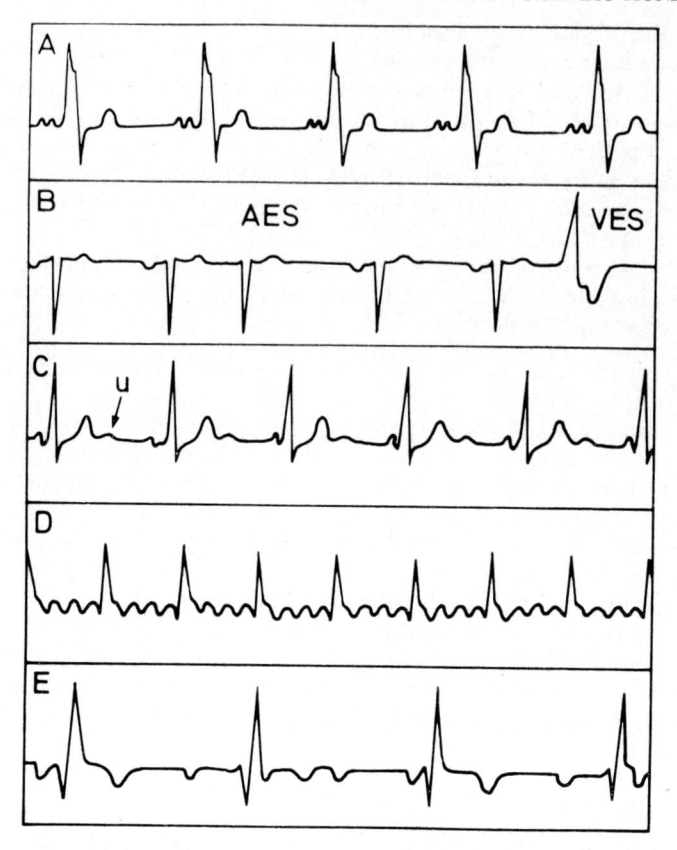

ECG 21. (A) sinus rhythm at normal heart rate; (B) extrasystole (atrial, AES; ventricular, VES); (C) U wave; (D) atrial flutter; (E) complete heart block.

  (a) Atrial—identical to normal QRS–T complexes,
  (b) Ventricular—different configuration to normal QRS–T complexes.

Alternatively the extra feature may be small and rounded:
  (a) U wave—just after the T wave (can look very like an extra P wave),
  (b) extra P wave
    if heart rate is slow—arrhythmia is probably heart block,
    if heart rate is fast—arrhythmia is probably atrial flutter

Note: Extra T waves alone (i.e. without QRS) do not occur.

MONITOR OBSERVATION 59

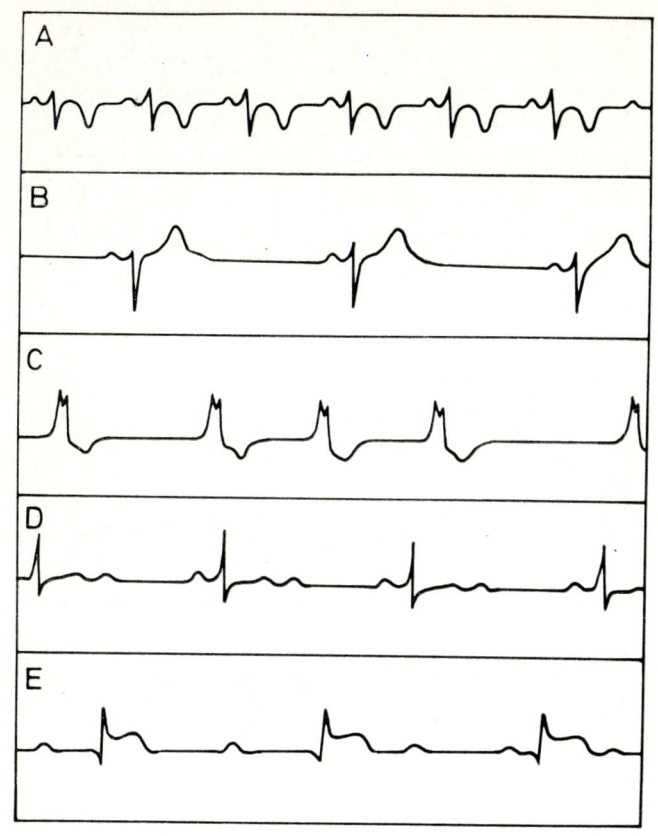

ECG 22. (A) sinus rhythm at normal heart rate; (B)–(E) slow heart rates; (B) sinus brachycardia; (C) slow atrial fibrillation; (D) second degree heart block; (E) complete heart block.

10. Slow Heart Rate (Bradycardia) (ECG 22B–E)

Large distance between spikes of successive QRS–T complexes. Check and confirm bradycardia by taking the pulse. The causes may be:

(a) Sinus brachycardia (slow normal rhythm) — Slow but otherwise normal trace.

(b) Slow atrial fibrillation — No P waves, rate irregular.

(c) Some form of heart block — Extra P waves. Inspect P–R segment carefully to assess whether it is normal, prolonged or varying in its length.

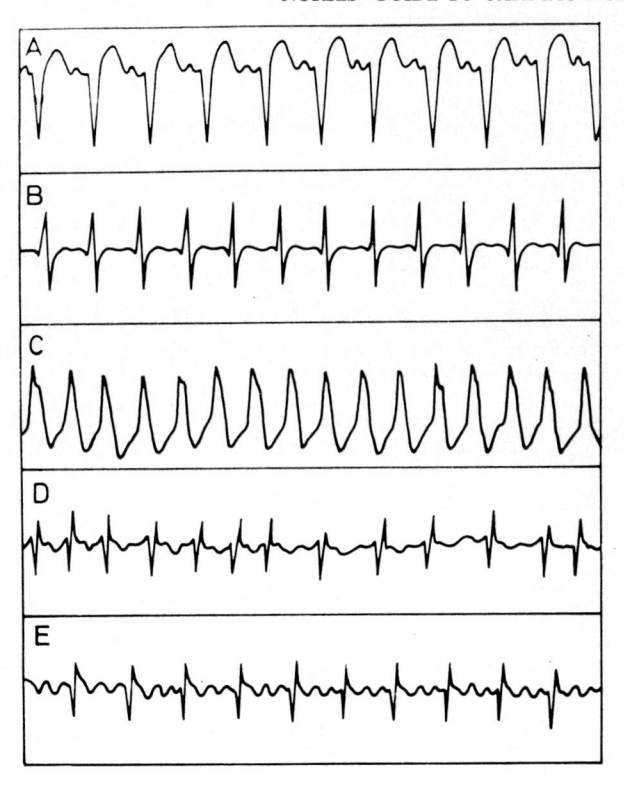

ECG 23. (A)–(E) fast heart rates; (A) sinus tachycardia; (B) atrial tachycardia; (C) ventricular tachycardia; (D) rapid atrial fibrillation; (E) atrial flutter.

11. Fast Heart Rate (Tachycardia) (ECG 23A–E)

Short distance between spikes of successive QRS–T complexes. Check and confirm presence of tachycardia by taking the pulse. Differentiation of the cause of the tachycardia, may be difficult. The causes may be:

	P waves	Configuration of QRS–T complexes	Heart rate
(a) Sinus tachycardia (fast normal rhythm)	Present	Normal	Regular
(b) Atrial tachycardia	Absent	Normal	Regular

	P waves	*Configuration of QRS–T complexes*	*Heart rate*
(c) Ventricular tachycardia	Absent	Large, wide	Regular
(d) Rapid atrial fibrillation	Absent	Normal	Irregular
(e) Atrial flutter	Extra P waves	Normal	Regular, occasionally irregular

Index

A–C interference 57
Acetone, for skin cleaning 10
Acidosis, after cardiac arrest 43
Adrenaline 12
Alarm system on cardiac monitor 4
Alcohol for skin cleaning 9
Angina 29
Arrhythmias 1, 2, 15, 19–44
Atria 12, 13
Atrial contraction 12, 13, 30, 33, 37, 38
Atrial extrasystole 23, 25, 26, 29, 58
Atrial fibrillation (AF) 26, 33–34, 59, 61
   significance 34
Atrial flutter 30, 31, 40–42, 58, 61
   significance 32
Atrial relaxation 14
Atrial tachycardia 29, 30, 31, 60
   significance 29
Atrio-ventricular (AV) node 12, 25
Atrium 11
Atropine 20, 42, 45
Attacks, Stokes–Adams 42, 45
AV node 12, 25

Base-line wandering 57
Blood pressure, fall of 20, 29, 32, 42, 45
Breathlessness 42, 45
Brightness of monitor screens 5
Bundle of His 12, 13
   bundle branches 13
Bradycardia 59
   sinus 19–21

Cardiac apex 33
Cardiac arrest 1, 2, 42, 43–44, 55
Cardiac asystole 42, 43–44, 45, 55
Cardiac catheterization 2
Cardiac massage 43

Cardiac monitor observation 14–17, 47, 55–61
Cardiac monitoring
   aim 1
   components 2
   indications 2
Cardiac pacing 42, 43, 44, 45–54
   components 45
   disturbances of
     competition (extrasystoles) 51
     loss of pacing impulse 47
     weak pacing impulse 49
   monitor observation 47
Cardiac surgery 1, 2, 27, 32, 42
Carotid sinus massage 30
Catheter electrode 45
Catheterization, cardiac 2
Channel selection 5
Chest electrodes 8–10, 57
   application 9–10
   position 9
Circulation, anatomy of 11
Cleaning, skin 9–10, 57
Competition 51
Complete heart block (CHB) 37–40, 42, 45
   and extrasystoles 42
Configuration, of wave 14, 55
Consciousness, loss of 20, 42, 43
Controls of monitor 4
Coupling 25

Demand pacemaker 54
Diastole 33
Digitalis 34
   toxicity 25, 27, 42
Digoxin 34
Dilated pupils (cardiac arrest) 42, 43
Diptheria 42
Diuretics 27

ECG oscilloscope 2–5
  indications 2
ECG trace, normal 13–16
  abnormal 55–61
  'fuzzy' 10, 56–57
  spikey 57
  wandering base-line 57
Ectopic beat (see also Extrasystole) 21–27
Electrode
  for monitoring 2, 7–10
    chest 8–9
    limb 7
    replacement 10
  for cardiac pacing 45
    catheter 45
    skin or indifferent 45
  jelly 10
Electrolyte disturbances 27
Ether, for skin cleaning 9
Ether-meths, for skin cleaning 9
Extra P wave 15, 31, 36, 39, 40, 58
Extra QRS–T complex 15, 22, 50, 58
Extrasystole 21–27
  atrial 23, 25, 26, 29, 58
  coupling 25
  nodal 25
  supraventricular 25
  ventricular 23–25, 58
    after myocardial infarction 26, 44
    multifocal 27
    with cardiac pacing 51
    with heart block 42

Fast heart rate (see also Tachycardia) 15, 60
Fibrillation
  atrial 26, 33–34, 59, 61
  ventricular 30, 42, 45, 53
  waves 33
First degree heart block 35
Flutter
  atrial 30, 31, 40–42, 58, 61
  ventricular 43
Functional heart block 31, 34, 41
'Fuzzy' trace 5, 10, 56–57

Haemorrhage 21
Heart, anatomy 11

Heart beat indicator 4
Heart block 35–42, 45, 58, 59
  complete (CHB) 37–40, 42, 45
  first degree 35
  functional 31, 34, 41
  recognition 40
  second degree 35–37, 40
  significance 42
  Wenckebach phenomenon 37, 40
  with extrasystoles 42
Heart disease 14
  and extrasystoles 27
Heart failure
  acute 21
  and arrhythmias 29, 32, 34, 42, 45
Heart muscle 12–13
Heart rate 15
  fast 15, 60
  irregular 15, 33, 36, 49–51, 61
  slow 15, 59
Heart surgery
  and arrhythmias 27, 32, 42
  and monitoring 1, 2
Hypokalaemia 27
Hypotension 20, 29, 32. 34, 42, 45

Impulse
  cardiac 12, 19, 29, 35
  pacing 45, 47, 49, 50, 52, 53, 54
Indicator, of heart beat 4
Indifferent electrode 45
Interference pattern 10, 56–57
Irritation of skin 10
Isoprenaline 42, 45

Jelly, electrode 10

Leads, of patient cable 4
Lignocaine 27
Limb electrodes 7, 57
  application 9–10
Loss of consciousness 20, 42, 43

Mains cable 3
Micropore tape 10
Mitral stenosis 34

INDEX

Monitor (cardiac) 1
  components 2–4
  observation 14–17, 47, 55–61
Morphine 20
'Multifocal' ventricular extrasystoles 27
Muscle, heart 12–13, 25
Myocardial infarction 1, 2, 20, 21, 26, 32, 34, 42, 52, 54

'Nodal' extrasystole 25

P wave 13, 14, 45
  absence of 29, 33
  extra 15, 31, 36, 39, 40, 58
  saw tooth 31
Pacemaker
  for cardiac pacing 1, 2, 45, 54
  of heart 13, 37
Pacing, cardiac 45–54
  components 45
  disturbances of 47, 49–51
  indications for 45
  monitor observation 47
Pacing electrodes 45, 46
Pacing impulse (PI) 45
  extra PI 50, 51
  loss of PI 47
  weak PI 49
Patient cable 4
Patient observation 1, 15, 55
Pethidine 20
Pneumonia 34
Potassium deficiency 27
P–R segment 13
  'apparent' 40
  prolonged 35
  varying 37, 38, 39
Premature ventricular
  beat (PVB) 21
  contraction (PVC) 21
Pulse deficit 33
Pulse rate 16, 59, 60
Pulselessness 42, 43
Purkinje fibres 12

QRS complex 13–14
  increased width of 25, 29

QRS–T complex 14, 16, 45
  dropped 37, 40, 49
  extra 15, 22, 58

Ratemeter 4
Record system 4
Rheumatic fever 42
Rheumatic heart disease 34
Rules, for monitor observation 14

SA node 12, 13, 29, 33
Salvos (ventricular extrasystoles) 27
Second degree heart block 35–37, 40–42
Selector switch 4
Serum potassium, low 27
Signals, alarm on cardiac monitor 4
Sino-atrial (SA) node 12, 13, 29, 33
Sinus bradycardia 19–21, 59
  significance 20
Sinus rhythm 13, 16–17, 53, 54
Sinus tachycardia 19–21, 60
  significance 20
Skin
  cleaning for electrode application 9–10
  electrode for cardiac pacing 45
  grease removal 10
  irritation 10
Slow heart rate (*see also* Bradycardia) 15, 59
Smoking, and extrasystoles 27
Sodium bicarbonate 44
Spikey trace 57
S–T segment 14
Stokes–Adams attacks 42, 45
'Supraventricular' extrasystole 25
Sympathetic stimulation 12

T wave 13, 14, 58
Tachycardia 60
  atrial 29–30, 60
  sinus 19–21, 60
  ventricular 29–30, 42, 45, 53, 61
Thyrotoxicosis 21, 34
Trace ECG 13
  'fuzzy' 10, 56–57
  spikey 57
  wandering base-line 57

'U' wave 14, 58

Vagus nerve 12, 20
Valve, heart 11
Vasovagal attack 20
Ventricular
  contraction 13
    premature 21
  extrasystole 23–25, 58
    after myocardial infarction 26, 44
    multifocal 27
    with cardiac pacing 51
    with heart block 42
  fibrillation 30, 42, 45, 53
  flutter 43
  muscle 12, 13
  pacemaker 37

Ventricular (*cont.*)
  relaxation 13
  tachycardia 29–30, 42, 45, 53, 61
    significance 29
Visual alarm signals 4

Wandering base-line 57
Wave
  extra 58
  P 13–14, 29, 31, 33, 36, 40, 45, 58
  T 13–14, 58
  U 14, 58
Wenckebach phenomenon 37–40

X-ray screening 45